TOTAL FITNESS FOR MEN

TOTAL FITNESS FOR MEN

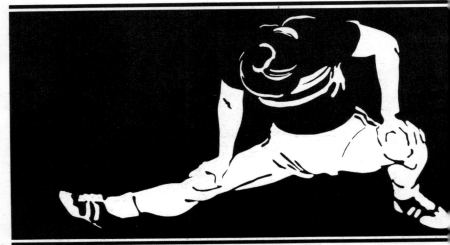

J. TILLMAN HALL
University of Southern California

GOODYEAR PHYSICAL ACTIVITIES SERIES
EDITED BY J. TILLMAN HALL

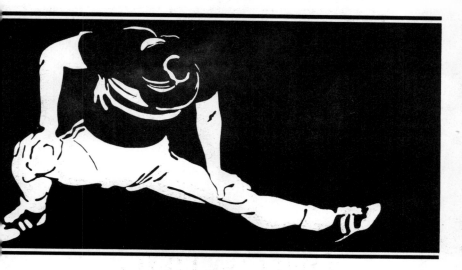

GOODYEAR PUBLISHING COMPANY, INC.
Santa Monica, California 90401

Library of Congress Cataloging in Publication Data

Hall, J Tillman.
  Total fitness for men.

  (Goodyear physical activities series)
  Bibliography: p. 86
  1. Physical fitness.   2. Physical fitness—Testing.
  3. Exercise.   I. Title.
  GV436.H26   613.7′044   79-22842
  ISBN 0-8302-9110-5

TOTAL FITNESS FOR MEN
J. Tillman Hall

Current printing (last digit):
10 9 8 7 6 5 4 3 2 1
Y-9110-1
Printed in the United States of America

ACKNOWLEDGMENTS

For their help with the pictures, special thanks are extended to:

Sergej de Duvillard
Bob Gerandola
Sarah Ingber
Jerry Kelly
Toshio Moritani
Lyn Sheffield

Special appreciation to Madalynne Lewis for her editing and typing of the manuscript.

CONTENTS

BIOGRAPHY

J. Tillman Hall has written or edited over 30 books on education and physical education.

He began his career in Big Sandy, Tennessee, as principal of the elementary school and head coach of sports at the high school. After a stint in the Navy during World War II, he became coach and Head of the Physical Education Department at Pepperdine University. He later moved to his present position of Professor and Head of the Physical Education Department at the University of Southern California.

Dr. Hall holds an Ed.D. degree from the University of Southern California. He is a recipient of the National Honor Award of the American Alliance for Health, Physical Education, Recreation, and Dance, and is listed in *Who's Who in the United States*.

DEDICATION

In Memory of

Travis and Kirk Hall
Frank and Willa Babb

They asked little for themselves but gained unusual
contentment by helping others.

EDITOR'S NOTE

Goodyear Publishing Company is pleased to add TOTAL FITNESS FOR MEN, a guide to healthy living, to its Physical Activities Series. This book examines all the facets of fitness: exercise, endurance and strength, nutrition and weight control. The book opens with a discussion of the major and submajor components of fitness (endurance, strength and flexibility are the major components; power, coordination and reaction time are the submajor components) and gives the reader exercises that will increase his capacity in each area. These exercises are clearly demonstrated in over 60 photographs which portray the specific exercise needed to accomplish a specific goal.

Next the reader is given a Physical Fitness Profile Chart to record and evaluate weight, size and fitness deviations.

Information about preconditioning, nutrition, weight control, and the development and maintenance of a symmetrical posture further equip him with the tools necessary for achieving total fitness.

The guiding theory behind this book is, what you don't use, you loose. Physical activity is not only important for health maintenance, but can be a satisfying dimension of life that has mental and emotional benefits. In the Chapter, "There's Another Way" emphasis has been placed on the benefits of engaging in a lifetime sport to keep fit so that artificial exercise programs can be kept to a minimum.

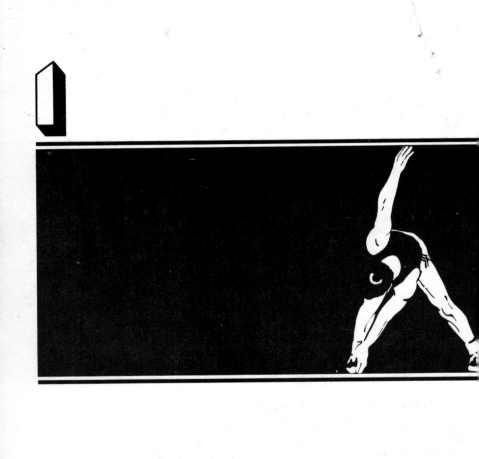

INTRODUCTION

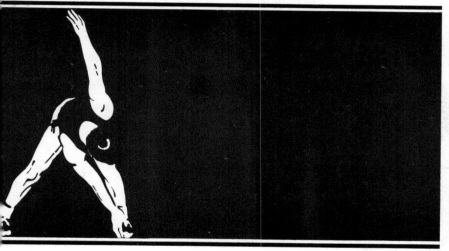

░NTEGRATED EFFECTIVENESS

To have "integrated effectiveness" means having the emotional, mental, spiritual, social, and physical attributes that are considered essential to achieve self-actualization. Your ultimate aim should be to strive for total development by making a continuous effort to develop your maximum potential. Total fitness may be virtually impossible, but we should always be progressing toward this goal.

No two living organisms are exactly alike, and so prescribing selective experiences for total fitness would be an extraordinarily complicated assignment. However, renowned educators have repeatedly stated that physically conditioned people tend to be well adjusted both socially and psychologically. Since the mind and the body have a profound influence on each other, the acquisition of cognitive, behavioral, and movement skills contributes to total effectiveness.

Through a discretionary selection of experiences you can acquire knowledge and skills that will help you approach total fitness. Without physical fitness you cannot achieve integrated effectiveness. Unless you have severe physical limitations, you *can* improve your physical-fitness profile. However, genetic differences will make the conditioning process more difficult for some than for others, but anyone who makes the effort is assured of making progress. It requires a personal commitment—no one else can achieve fitness for you. The question is, how fit do you want to be? What price are you willing to pay?

Too often, physical-fitness enthusiasts suggest that anything less than maximal fitness is unimportant; this is too bad. Research has not verified that health benefits increase for those who have attained more than 50 percent of their physical-fitness potential. However, this leaves plenty of room for improvement, since it is doubtful that the average person has achieved even 10 percent of this quota, which is substantially below the level everyone should try to maintain. Not to achieve a better fitness quota is extremely risky, somewhat like driving on the freeway with less than a gallon of gas and deflated tires in rush-hour traffic.

In 1900 some 75 percent of the people living in the United States resided in rural areas. Most were engaged in arduous manual labor, which in many ways contributed towards the development of certain physical-fitness components. Today over 75 percent of the population lives in cities, where technological advancements have virtually eliminated employment that requires the use of big muscles. We have become accustomed to a push-button, power-steering, ten-speed lifestyle. Thermostats that automatically activate switches controlling furnaces, refrigerators, and air conditioners, are found in nearly all of our homes. In fact, for most of us, neither our professional work nor our household chores help much in developing or maintaining physical fitness. The popularization of work-saving gadgets has eliminated hours of drudgery but at the same time has reduced, for most people, the optimum level of fitness. Without significant big-muscle activity, optimal fitness is not possible. It is assumed that if the positive effects of exercise are understood, you will want to be more active; knowledge is necessary for wise self-direction, but unless it changes your behavior its value is minimal.

COMPONENTS OF PHYSICAL FITNESS

The term physical fitness means having the ability to function at your very best. Physical fitness is a personal attribute influenced by a number of individual factors, including heredity and environment. Research reveals that it is transitory and will disappear unless maintained through vigorous exercise.

From a scientific viewpoint, the components of physical fitness may be divided into major and submajor categories. Those components considered most fundamental are endurance, strength, and flexibility. The submajor categories are essential for skillful movements but have an indirect relationship to total fitness. These components are coordination, power, reaction time, and good body mechanics.

1. Endurance.

Endurance is sometimes referred to as stamina; it is the ability to withstand fatigue, hardship, or stress. The two types of endurance most frequently mentioned in physical-fitness literature are cardiovascular and muscular. Both may be achieved at the same time through participation in appropriately selected activities.

Research indicates the need to maintain a heart rate in excess of 50 percent of maximum capacity for more than five minutes at at time, to improve cardiovascular endurance. Activities that require continuous vigorous movement, such as running, badminton, racquetball, handball, basketball, bicycling, swimming, folk dancing, and mountain climbing, will help improve both cardiovascular and muscular endurance. Sustained interest in exercise usually results from taking part in sports with others. The more skilled you become, the more you seem to enjoy vigorous exercise. A daily 15 to 18 minute two-mile run would build adequate cardiovascular endurance. It would require at least an hour's participation in a vigorous sport every day to achieve the same results. Select your activity; the choice is yours.

Cardiorespiratory recovery. This is the speed with which the heartbeat and respiration rate return to normal after exercise. The cardiorespiratory system includes heart, lungs, blood, and blood vessels. Their condition and how they function is the greatest determiner of physical fitness.

The heart.

This is the primary organ in the body. It is first to initiate life and the last to retain it before the onset of rigor mortis. Physical fitness would be impossible without a well-conditioned heart.

The heart is a powerful muscle about the size of a clenched fist, and is responsible for pumping some five to six quarts of blood throughout the body every minute. This pumping process may increase five to eight times during exercise.

The principal pacemaker, the sinoatrial (SA) node, and the secondary pacemaker, the atrioventricular (AV) node, initiate an impulse that causes the heart muscle to contract some 72 times per minute, 4,320 times per hour, or about 103,680 times each day. Vigorous exercise may more than double the number of contractions per minute, and spread over a prolonged period, tends to increase the heart's size. Cardiac hypertrophy, sometimes referred to as "athlete's heart," has a number of advantages. It can contract less frequently but more forcefully, thus operating with greater efficiency.

The development of cardiovascular endurance depends on the frequency and intensity of training sessions. An increased workload that elevates the heart to 50 percent of its maximum capacity eight to ten minutes per day would improve cardiovascular endurance. Less exercise would probably do little more than maintain the status quo.

Respiratory function.

Any functional deficiency in this system will inhibit physical fitness.

When oxygen uptake is sufficient to meet the consumption rate of all tissues in the body, it is classified as *aerobic* activity. Vigorous exercise on a regular basis may increase aerobic capacity some 25 percent. The primary purpose for aerobic exercise, then, is to increase cardiorespiratory endurance, and exercise chosen by most adults seems to fit within this classification.

When the oxygen supply is insufficient to meet the tissue needs it is referred to as *anaerobic*. In short bouts of exercise such as sprints, and during the initial stages of other vigorous activities, one may run up an oxygen debt; for most adults the value of anaerobic exercise is questionable.

The blood and blood vessels.

The cardiovascular system includes the heart, arteries and blood. The development of strong skeletal muscles through exercise usually results in a strong cardiovascular system.

2. Strength.

The physical power generated through muscular contraction is indicative of strength. When muscles are challenged by use of the "overload principle" they become stronger, and are consequently capable of a greater workload.

Isotonic (dynamic muscle training) and *isometric* (static muscle training) are the two most often described methods of improving strength. Dynamic muscle training involves movement exercise such as weight lifting, throwing, striking, and running. Frequency and intensity are important factors in using this method to develop strength. Static muscle training involves minimal shortening of the muscle fibers. Applying force against an immovable object, such as trying to lift a 1,000-pound weight, characterizes this type of strength development.

The controversy over these two methods of strength training has not been resolved. Experiments with matched groups using both isotonic and isometric exercise failed to prove one method better than the other. However, it is generally agreed that it requires less time to use isometrics for strength development, although most people prefer isotonic exercise.

3. Flexibility.

Flexibility refers to motion that is unrestricted through the normal range of movement. It is the ability to bend, twist, or turn without breaking. Infrequent stretching, twisting, and rotating of major body segments results in the loss of suppleness. Flexibility can be achieved by forcibly flexing and extending the muscles and connective tissues through a complete range of motion. An appropriately designed calisthenic program will provide exercises for this component of physical fitness.

4. Coordination and Agility.

Coordination is the harmonious functioning of a muscle or group of muscles in the execution of a complex task. Without coordination you would most likely experience considerable embarrassment when participating in competitive sports. It is important to continuously attempt to refine your movement patterns. A highly coordinated person has developed maximum control of both the synergistic (working) and antagonistic (resting) muscles; this includes control over the central nervous system and the reflex arc (involuntary movement), as well as a kinesthetic awareness of the autonomic (self-controlling) system. Thus both voluntary and involuntary muscle movements are sensitized in a coordinated person.

Agility refers to alertness, quickness, and nimble-ness. A skillful performer will usually have all of these.

Balance is the ability to achieve a position between extremes and still maintain equilibrium. The well-coordinated person must be concerned with both static (stationary) and dynamic (moving) balance. Static balance is essential in assuming the ready position prior to such movement patterns as those needed to bat, run, and field in baseball; dive competitively; make the center snap in football; and begin most running events in track. Without dynamic balance, intricate movement patterns in sports would be impossible. Complicated movement patterns involving multiple postures require equibalanced muscular control.

5. Power.

Power is the force that you are capable of exerting. For calculation purposes, researchers speak of units of energy per second, or foot-pounds per second. Traditionally, power was expressed in terms of horsepower, with one horsepower the equivalent of 550 foot-pounds per second. For our purposes, it may be measured by the force one person can exert in a unit of time.

6. Reaction Time.

The speed or quickness with which a person can move one or more parts of his body is known as reaction time. The ability to move quickly is a hereditary characteristic and can best be improved through a readiness for action and refinement of biomechanical techniques. Although it is possible to improve your strength, endurance, and flexibility by 50 percent, your reaction time can be improved only 8 to 10 percent. However, to be successful in competitive sports requires the best reaction time possible—and it *can* be improved.

7. Motor Skills.

From a biological viewpoint there is some difficulty in classifying movement efficiency as a component of physical fitness. Nevertheless, significant motor skills are a part of total fitness. Without the development of kinesthetic sensations, locomotor movement patterns would be erratic. Motor skills, which are basic to any activity in which we participate, are based upon certain principles of body mechanics that occur as a person grows and develops. Of course, there are certain physical, mental, and emotional factors involved too. In general, we think of motor skills as a sequence of learned movement patterns including readying (physical conditioning), learning (practice for quantity), perfecting (practice for quality), and retaining (skill maintenance). If you can engage in persistent activity requiring a vigorous motor skill you have achieved cardiovascular endurance.

DIET AND EXERCISE

Another aspect of physical fitness which cannot be ignored is nutrition and weight control. Most Americans are overweight, many are malnourished, and some are both!

The truth is, the body's needs are simple but specific: We need *proteins* to build and maintain body cells; *carbohydrates* to supply energy for work and play; and *fats* for energy and insulation. *Vitamins* and *minerals* are necessary in small amounts to regulate metabolism and normal growth and functioning. Without a proper balance of these basic nutrients, our bodies would undergo undesirable changes.

If your daily diet contains excessive carbohydrates

and fats you are likely to gain weight. Weight is influenced by heredity and metabolism, but it can be nutritionally controlled when combined with selective exercise. In most cases, overweight is simply due to overeating. If his food intake were carefully chosen, the average American could reduce the amount he eats by approximately 50 percent and feel much better.

Most people agree that exercising regularly makes them feel better, too. In fact, I have never heard anyone voice any other opinion. This good feeling is extremely difficult to understand completely. Exercise apparently stimulates body cells, thereby producing a general tuning of the entire organism. This tends to enhance the optimal functioning of movement patterns which are in turn conducive to pleasurable sensations. In other words, exercise adds zest to life! If you have not experienced this zest, try it—you'll like it!

A number of experimental studies reported in *Research Quarterly, Physical Fitness Research Digest,* and *Exercise and Sport Science Reviews* describe the benefits received from participating in various exercise programs. Some of these studies will be referred to later in this book. In general, the research indicates that exercise enhances the participant's physical, social, emotional, and economic life style. Furthermore, people in good physical condition tend to recuperate more rapidly from illness or accidents.

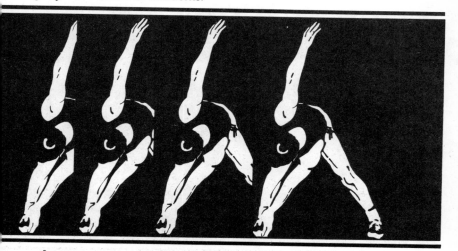

It is important, when striving for high-level physical fitness, to begin with a thorough physical examination. This is especially true for anyone who is recovering from illness or who has been inactive for a long time.

The body you have is the one you are stuck with—for life! It is very durable, can recover from considerable abuse, and—when intelligently used and maintained—will function efficiently and effectively for many years. It stands to reason that the more you know about the body's composition and its proper use, the more you know about how you should live. The choice is yours. Informed people know the importance of a regular physical exercise program.

2

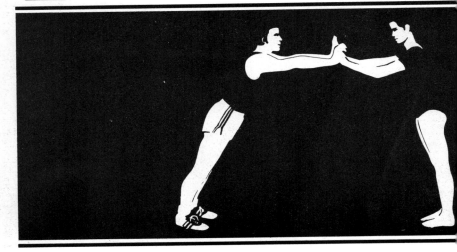

ENDURANCE, STRENGTH, & FLEXIBILITY

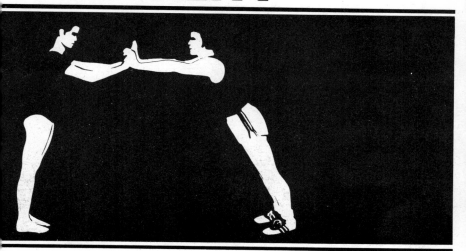

T here is little disagreement that *endurance, strength,* and *flexibility* are the major components of physical fitness. All three are extremely important and will be discussed in greater detail in this chapter.

The three types of endurance most frequently discussed in physical fitness literature are cardiovascular, muscular, and respiratory endurance. Each implies the ability to withstand fatigue, hardship, and stress.

CARDIOVASCULAR ENDURANCE

The cardiovascular system includes the heart, arteries, capillaries, veins, and the blood. Prolonged activity requires cardiovascular endurance, and is based on the ability to withstand the stress placed on the entire system. Continued stress produces a baffling syndrome called fatigue. Once this begins there is a feeling of inadequacy associated with the desire to rest.

The heart.

Since the heart is the most important organ in the body, let us review some of its most important characteristics. The heart is a muscular organ about the size of a clenched fist and pumps some ten pints of blood through more than 1,000 complete circuits, thus actually pumping 5,000 to 6,000 quarts of blood per day. In fact, these five to six quarts of blood are forced each minute

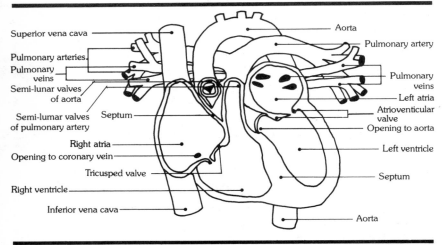

Figure 2.1   *The human heart*

through some 60,000 miles of arteries, capillaries, and veins. During vigorous exercise the velocity of the blood may increase some five to ten times over that which exists when the body is at rest.

The heart weighs less than a pound, is cone-shaped like the popular Valentine image, and lies obliquely in the chest cavity near the mid-center body line. Its walls are composed of thick, striated, muscle fibers twisted into rings, whorls, and loops. It is composed of a double pump system, which is necessary for maintaining blood velocity. (See Figure 2.1.)

Chambers. The human heart is divided into four chambers: *left* and *right atria* and the *left* and *right ventricles*. Blood laden with carbon dioxide from the *vena cava* and *coronary sinus* empties into the right atrium. Blood rich in oxygen from the *pulmonary veins* empties into the left atrium. The ventricles are the pumping chambers of the heart. Nonoxygenated blood is handled by the right ventricle and oxygenated blood by the left ventricle.

Valves. Two types of appropriately placed valves, the *atrioventricular* and the *semilunar,* prevent blood from leaking back into the heart. Anything that interferes with the "fit" of these valves, such as scarring, shortening, or thickening, may interfere with circulatory-system efficiency. Damaged heart valves sometimes limit both the quality and the quantity of life.

Pacemaker. The *sinoatrial node* (SA), an area of specialized tissue in the right atrium, is recognized as the principle *pacemaker.* If for some reason the SA node does not function, the *atrioventricular node* (AV) takes over the initiation of the beat.

Cardiac cycle. The *cardiac cycle* is composed of three phases, which occur as follows:

1. Atrial systole (both atria contract), creating the sound *lub*.

2. Ventricular systole (both ventricles contract), creating the sound *dub*.

3. Diastole (whole heart is relaxed), creating a pause. Extra sounds, such as excessive turbulence and regurgitation of the blood, are indicative of defects in the valves and are audible with a stethoscope.

Blood.

Blood is actually a fluid form of connective tissue, pumped by the heart throughout the circulatory vessels. It is composed of red blood cells, white blood cells, platelets, and plasma. Having too much or too little of any of these elements affects the functioning of the entire system. The five or six quarts of blood each person has acts as a coolant and as a transport medium whereby gases, hormones, and nutrients are brought to every cell.

At the same time waste products are moved to elimination stations. The red blood cells transport oxygen and carbon dioxide between the tissues and the lungs. The white blood cells defend the body against infection. Platelets aid in the repair of damaged vessels. Plasma, a waterlike substance that makes up 50 percent of the blood, acts as a coolant, transports all blood cells and nutrients and has viscosity about twice that of water. The blood cells and platelets are formed in the red bone marrow. The extent to which exercise aids cell production is not precisely known, but it is believed to be influential.

Blood vessels. Arteries carry blood from the heart to the capillaries, which empty into the veins, and they return the blood to the heart. If all the blood vessels in one adult were hooked up end to end, they would extend thousands of miles.

Arteries differ in size, and in the structure of their walls, and in their function. Some are elastic and some are muscular; others, called arterioles, function in a distributory capacity. Proper functioning of the arteries depends upon their extensibility and elasticity. The aorta and pulmonary arteries measure 1¼ inches in diameter at their origin, while the diameter of arterioles is less than that of a single hair.

Ateriolés are so small that blood cells have to pass through them in single file, and in many parts of the body these vessels lie so close together that a needle point cannot be inserted between them without damaging the capillary wall. Vasomotor nerve fibers provide stimuli to the muscle tissue in the walls of the blood vessels. These fibers are divided into two sets: vasoconstrictor and vasodilator nerves. Exercise conditions the muscles in the walls of the circulatory vessels along with those in surrounding areas. Without this conditioning, blood vessels would probably lose some of their elasticity.

Cardiovascular Diseases.

Cardiovascular disease and insufficiency are responsible for over 60 percent of all deaths in the United States. Everyone should be knowledgeable about the number-one killer and what might possibly be done to avoid a heart seizure.

1. *Atherosclerosis*—thickening or buildup of fatty deposits in the blood vessels; probably begins before one becomes of age. Recommended prevention: diet— avoid obesity, keep blood pressure down, cut down on cigarettes, exercise regularly.

2. *Angina Pectoris*—pain from oxygen deprivation. Recommended prevention: diet, reduce activity, reduce stress.

3. *Heart failure*—may be due to improper functioning; high blood pressure, defective heart valves, disease, poison, or damaged heart muscle. Recommended prevention: regular health examination, diet, exercise.

4. *Cardiac arrest*—heart stops; may be due to heart attack, strangulation, drowning, or electrocution. Treatment: immediate medical attention, resuscitation—must start circulation within three to four minutes.

5. *Rheumatic condition*—inflammation of connective tissues that scars heart muscle and heart valves; occurs mostly during childhood. Treatment: penicillin.

6. *Congenital heart defects*—hole in septum separating chambers of the heart. Treatment: open-heart surgery.

7. *Strokes*—uncontrolled bleeding of blood vessels in the brain. Treatment: pray; and hope the bleeding is minimal, and stops.

8. *High blood pressure*—sustained constriction of blood vessels. Treatment: reduce weight if obese; rest, relax, see doctor, exercise regularly.

Efficiency of the Heart.

There are a number of tests to discover how well the heart functions. It is important to discover the effect of exercise upon the minute-volume and stroke-volume of the heart. To do this, special equipment (such as the *electrocardiograph*) is used to record the electric potentials associated with the electric currents that traverse the heart. Thus the electrocardiogram (EKG) is a valuable diagnostic research tool used to record the damage done by an obstruction of the vessels, and the exact location of a lesion.

1. Stress Test. Since a cursory health examination will not always reveal heart deficiencies, many exercise physiology laboratories have sophisticated electronic equipment with which maximal oxygen uptake can be measured. (Figure 2.2.) The results from this type of test are recognized as a reliable indicator of physical fitness.

2. Step Test. The Harvard Step Test, (Figure 2.3) developed during World War II, proved useful in classifying the fitness levels of young men. It not only

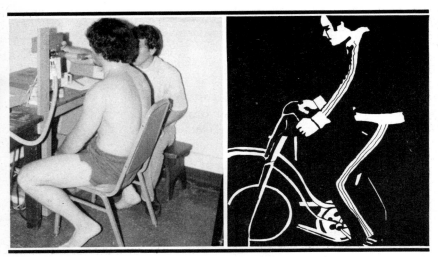

Figure 2.2 *Measuring aerobic capacity*

measures how much the heart rate rises during exercise, but how quickly it returns to its resting rate after exercise is concluded. The short-form test (see Chapter 4 for the larger form), as described by Mathews, is easy to administer. You need a 20-inch-high bench.

    a. Take standing resting heart rate.

    b. Step up-down, 30 steps per minute, for five minutes.

    c. Take 30-second pulse count one minute after the exercise.

$$INDEX = \frac{\text{seconds exercised} \times 100}{5.5 \times \text{pulse count}}$$

The average scores for the short forms were: below 50—poor; 50–80—average; above 80—good.

Another way to interpret the data would be to compute recovery to starting rate. If at the end of three minutes the heart beat is equal to or less than starting rate, it is excellent; 1 to 2 beats away, good; 3 to 4 beats away, fair; 5 to 6 beats away, poor; 7 beats away, very poor.

3. Field Test. Since most exercise laboratories are limited in size, with a minimal number of technicians and

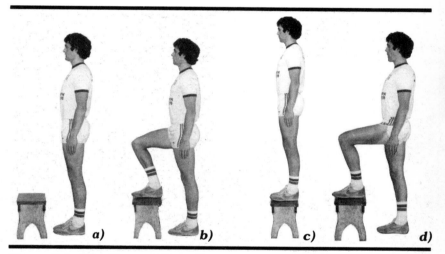

Figure 2.3 *The Harvard Step Test*

sophisticated equipment, some field tests have been devised that provide a fairly good measure of one's aerobic fitness. The 12 to 18 minute two-mile run is a pretty good indicator of fitness. The faster the time, the better the physical condition.

Through a physical-conditioning program, you can improve your cardiovascular fitness. As the workload increases there is a corresponding elevation of the heart rate, which enhances endurance. The training intensity should be at 55 to 65 percent of your maximum capacity for a minimum of 15 to 20 minutes at least three times a week for cardiovascular maintenance. More frequent and more intense training bouts would increase your endurance but it is doubtful if the effects would add any appreciable benefits.

Activities suitable for cardiovascular endurance training are jogging, basketball, racquetball, tennis, handball, volleyball, badminton, handball, mountain climbing, and vigorous dancing. The heart muscle, like the skeletal muscles, becomes stronger when it is vigorously exercised. The muscular walls of the arteries, veins and capillaries are also strengthened by exercise, thus improving the circulatory system's functioning process. Both *interval* training (work alternated with rest) and *continuous* training (lengthy exercise periods) have been used in developing cardiovascular endurance. *Circuit* training mixes running with other forms of exercise at various stations along the route.

MUSCULAR ENDURANCE

The human body is composed of some 650 to 700 separate muscles and they make up some 40 to 60 percent of its total weight. The muscles are divided into three types: skeletal, which are voluntary and propel the body; smooth, which form the walls of internal organs and blood vessels; and cardiac, which form the heart.

Muscle cannot push; they can only pull, and in doing so they shorten or contract. The skeletal muscles produce all the voluntary movements and are essential in the performance of many body functions. Muscle endurance cannot be achieved without intensive voluntary movement. Thus physical fitness requires locomotion as an instigator of the process. (See Figures 2.11, 2.12.)

Skeletal muscle action.

The skeletal muscles maintain posture, chew food, swallow, articulate speech, kiss girls, coordinate action; in other words, they are responsible for all volitional movement. All of these, plus numerous additional movements, require the development of muscle tissue.

Muscle tone.

Due to alternating nerve impulses, various groups of muscle fibers are stimulated, resulting in a partial contraction. This is muscle tone, which gives muscles a certain firmness as they pull upon their attachments. Muscle tone is present when the muscle reflexes and also when the muscle is relaxed and no action potential is induced, when its tone may be described as elastic.

Muscle structure.

Every skeletal muscle is composed of several bundles—fascicles—of muscle fibers. Each fascicle may contain up to 100 individual muscle fibers and is surrounded by a membrane called the *sarcolemma*. Each muscle group is enclosed in a sheet of fibrous tissue, the *fascia*. It is slippery, and so permits movement with minimal friction.

Muscle innervation.

Every skeletal muscle is supplied with one or more branches from larger nerve trunks, and the *efferent* nerve fibers terminate on muscle fibers near their center, the *motor end plate*. Muscle fibers are excitable, and when a stimulus is strong enough to produce a response the fibers will make a maximal contraction, the *all-or-non-law*. *Motor units* include all muscle fibers and nuerons in a single muscle bundle, and their actions are analyzed in describing muscle tonus and maintenance of posture.

Muscle contraction.

When muscle fibers receive a *threshold* stimulus, they contract. There are three processes to understand in muscular contraction:

1. *Neuromuscular,* the impulse transmitted from neuron to muscle fiber via motor end plate.

2. *Transmembrane,* the electrical charge distributed across the cell membrane; supports the all-or-none-theory.

3. *Sliding filament,* the myofilaments in the myofibrils in the muscle fibers which slide past each other when activated.

A single stimulus brings about a *single twitch,* which is the simplest contraction possible. The *Treppe Effect,* or "staircase" phenomena, occurs when a muscle receives a minimal stimulus three or four times per second. When a muscle contracts during exercise it is called an *isotonic* contraction. If the muscle is static during an effort it is referred to as an *isometric* contraction.

Experiments with matched groups using both isotonic and isometric exercise failed to prove one method better than the other in the development of physical fitness. It requires less time to benefit from isometric exercise, but most people prefer the game approach, isotonics, for their workout.

Groups of muscles working together to perform a task are called synergist. Those working in opposition are called *antagonist*. *Anti-gravity* muscles are those situated around joints, and through a steady contraction aid in the maintenance of posture. (See Figure 2.12.)

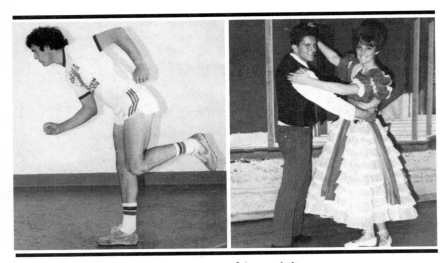

Figure 2.4 *Sprinting is an anaerobic activity.*
Figure 2.5 *Dancing is an aerobic activity.*

Both muscle soreness and fatigue resulting from exercise are chiefly due to the accumulation of lactic acid. Some soreness may be caused by small tears in the muscle fibers or in the connective tissue. Occasionally it may be due to a slight strain placed on the *flower-spray endings*, or delicate nerve terminations on the sarcolemma of a muscle spindle. The probable seats of fatigue are muscle fiber, motor end plates, motor nerve fibers, nerve cell body, and the *synapses*.

Muscular endurance can best be developed by using the *"overload principle."* Researchers agree that when a muscle is exercised regularly against gradually increasing resistance, both strength and muscle endurance will be enhanced. An increase in muscular endurance is associated with several factors. More fuel and oxygen are available, and there is an increase in muscle capillaries in regularly exercised muscles. Concomitant with these changes additional muscle fibers are activated.

RESPIRATORY ENDURANCE

The respiratory system includes the nose, trachea, pharynx, larynx, bronchii, and lungs. Its major

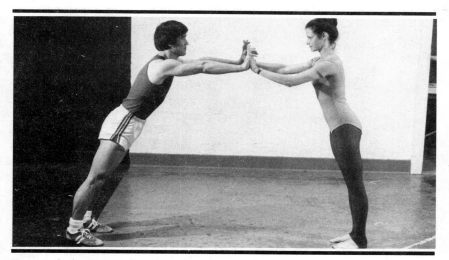

Figure 2.6 *Isometrics*

responsibilities are to bring oxygen into the lungs and to remove carbon dioxide from them.

The quantity of air expelled by a forcible exhalation after the deepest inhalation possible is called the *vital capacity*. This amounts to about 4000 cc (seven to eight pints) for an adult man. It is assumed that you can increase vital capacity through exercise.

During the continuous flow of blood through the capillaries of the lungs there is a diffusion of oxygen through the permeable membrane to the blood and of carbon dioxide from the blood.

Endurance, Strength & Flexibility   21

When the oxygen supply is insufficient it is termed *anaerobic*; when it is sufficient to meet the needs of all body tissues it is called *aerobic* fitness. In the sprints we run up an "oxygen debt," and it is called anaerobics (Figure 2.4), but when we play games, dance (Figure 2.5) or jog, we call it aerobics. The "second wind" syndrome appears to occur more frequently when engaged in anaerobics.

As the cardiovascular system is conditioned, so is the respiratory system. The immediate effects seem to be an increase in lung capacity, rate of breathing, and circulatory efficiency. A well conditioned person tends to breathe more economically, need less air, and suffer less

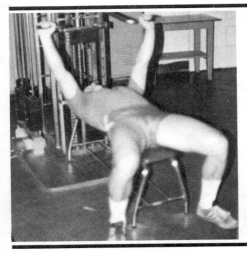

Figure 2.7 *Isotonics*

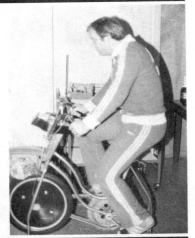

Figure 2.8 *Isokinetics*

stress from exercise than those who are less well conditioned. Maximum respiratory fitness may be reached in two to three months of vigorous training.

STRENGTH

Strength is the physical power generated through a summation of muscular contractions. It may be measured in three ways: *isometric,* power exerted against a nonmovable object; (Figure 2.6); *isotonic,* power exerted through a specific movement (Figure 2.7); and *isokinetic,* maximal contraction at a constant speed with accommodating resistance (Figure 2.8). Strength may be developed by any of these types of muscular contractions, or by a combination of all three. Furthermore, specific exercise may be selected so strength can be developed in one or more parts of the muscular system at the same time.

The exercises shown in Figures 2.6, 2.7 and 2.8 indicate how strength may be developed.

FLEXIBILITY

The third major component of physical fitness is *flexibility*. It represents the range of motion between the bones and other parts of the body. As we age, we tend to

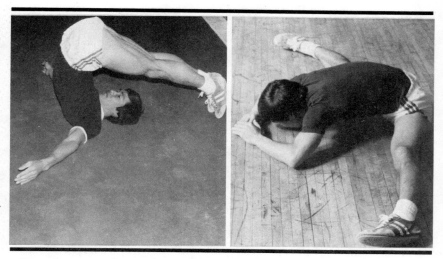

Figure 2.9 *Flexibility exercises*

lose our flexibility, which seems to be due to the shortening or loss of the connective tissues that surround the joints.

The range of motion can be increased by stretching the noncontractile tissues, such as the ligaments and tendons. By doing this, performance is improved in most physical activities. Both the develpment and maintenance of flexibility may be achieved through selected exercise that involves a full range of motion at each of the joints. Figure 2.9 shows examples of flexibility exercises.

Endurance, Strength & Flexibility   23

Movable Joints.

There are four major types of movement in the joints in the human body.

1. *Gliding.* Flexion and extension are brought about by sliding one bone over the surface of another, as happens in the knee joint.

2. *Angular.* This is an increase in the angle between one bone and another. The fingers and toes typify this kind of movement.

3. *Rotation.* This is a turning movement of a bone around an axis, such as is found in the elbow.

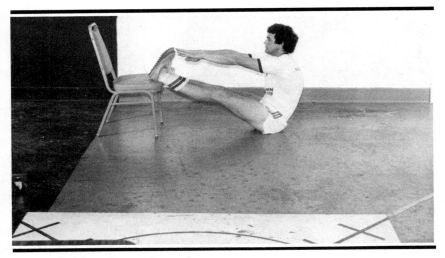

Figure 2.10a *Sit and reach*

4. *Circumduction.* This is the movement of a bone to circumscribe a conical space, such as the movement of a stretched-out leg or arm.

Due to numerous cultural, hereditary, and biological influences, the degree of flexibility tends to vary from one person to another, so you should not try to equal someone else's range of movement.

Instruments such as the *flexometer* have been developed to aid in determining joint flexibility. However, there are a number of commonly used classroom tests, techniques, and measurements. Some are shown in Figure 2.10. Leg lifts, equally valuable, are not shown.

After the range of movement has been identified for a given joint, it is not difficult to select exercise for both its maintenance and improvement. A high level of suppleness can be developed and maintained with selective exercise on a regular basis.

Endurance, strength, and flexibility are the major components of physical fitness. Unless we incorporate suitable activities into our lives, each of these components will slowly erode and become increasingly difficult to recapture. But by using the overload principle on a regular basis, age need only be a minimal deterrent in the maintenance of high-level fitness.

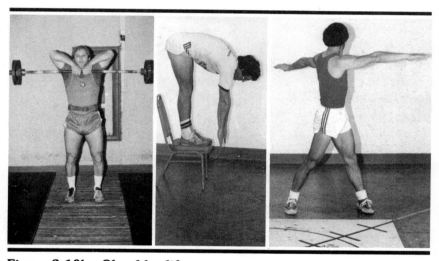

Figure 2.10b *Shoulder lift*
Figure 2.10c *Stand and reach*
Figure 2.10d *Arm rotation. Keep arms straight and rotate in small circles.*

MAJOR MUSCLES OF THE BODY

These major muscle groups make possible all physical movements. Your strength, stamina, skill, and economy of energy depend upon their teamwork. But their development depends on you. The best way to increase their ability is to increase their work load gradually. They need vigorous exercise—neither very light nor extremely strenuous —at regular intervals. Muscle developing activities include:

- running
- jumping
- throwing
- lifting
- pushing
- hitting
- stretching

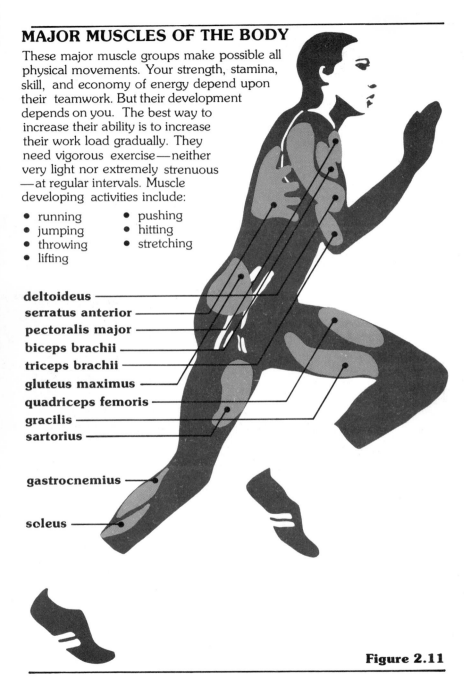

deltoideus
serratus anterior
pectoralis major
biceps brachii
triceps brachii
gluteus maximus
quadriceps femoris
gracilis
sartorius

gastrocnemius

soleus

Figure 2.11

ANTIGRAVITY MUSCLES

Six major groups of muscles work together to combat the pull of gravity and enable you to sit or stand upright. Muscles cannot push: they can only pull by contracting, or drawing their ends together. Vigorous exercise develops their strength and endurance. Mild exercise may be nearly useless.

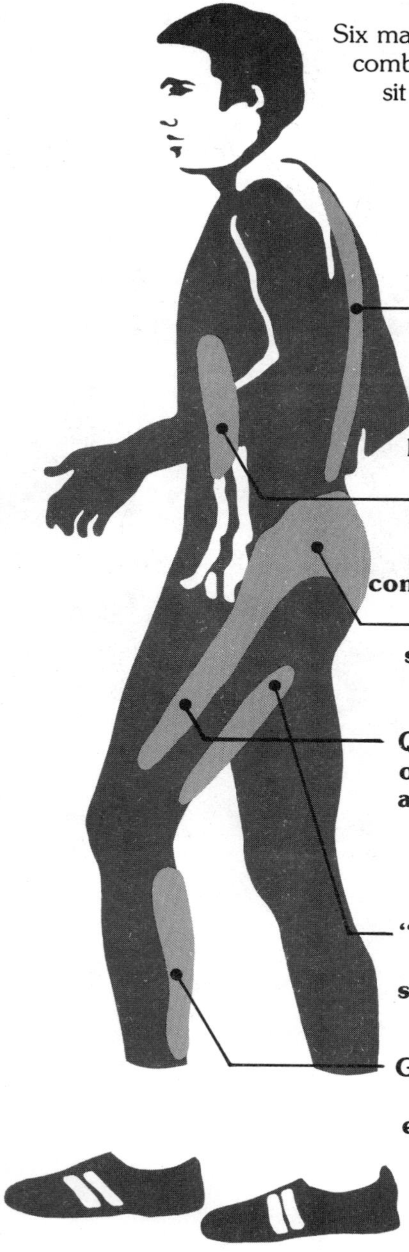

Trapezius (tra-pe'zi-us) latissimus (lat-is'i-mus) dorsi (dor'si) and sacrospinalis (sa'kro-spi-na'lis) muscles brace the back and shoulders and hold the vertebral column upright.

Obliquus (oblik'wus) transversus (trans-ver'sus) rectus (rek'tus) abdominis (ab-dom'i-nis) muscles contract and compress the abdomen.

Gluteus (glu'te-us) muscles support the floor of the pelvis and extend and rotate the femur.

Quadriceps (kwod'ri-seps) extensor or quadriceps femoris (fem-o'ris) is a four-headed muscle covering the front and sides of the thigh. It extends the thigh, and its rectus portion flexes it.

"Hamstrings"—The bicep denoris, somimembranosus and senitendinosus muscles extend the hip and flex the knee.

Gastrocnemius (gas-trok-ne'me-us) and soleus (so'le-us) muscles extend the foot and flex the lower part of the leg.

Figure 2.12

3

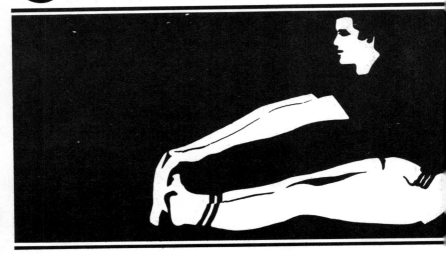

SUBMAJOR COMPONENTS OF PHYSICAL FITNESS

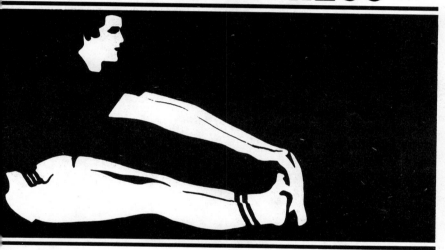

The submajor components that influence your physical fitness level are coordination, power, reaction time and body mechanics. These distinctive features do not have the same physiological importance in attaining physical fitness as endurance, strength, and flexibility, but they are extremely important if you wish to master motor skills.

COORDINATION

There is a harmonious interaction between groups of muscles, their origin and insertion, and the ligaments that help to hold the bones together at the joints. When this interaction takes place it produces coordination. Agility is produced by the interaction of the brain, spinal cord, and peripheral nerves. All voluntary movements are controlled in the motor area of the brain located in the *cerebral cortex*. The *cerebellum* controls balance, postural attitudes, and the adjustment of motor behavior. Repetitive skill drills until a desired movement pattern becomes automatic is the recommended procedure for the improvement of coordination. Maneuverability skills such as agility, balance, strength, speed, and flexibility may be sought separately or collectively. Whatever the choice, progression from the relatively simple to more complicated movement patterns seems to be the best

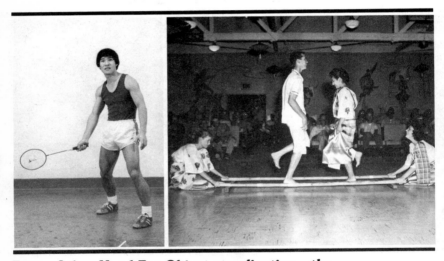

Figure 3.1a *Hand-Eye-Object coordination—the badminton volley.*
Figure 3.1b *Foot-Eye-Object coordination—Philipine Tinickling.*

procedure. It is easier to learn how to play one-wall rather than four-wall handball. Learning how to swing a lightweight tennis racquet is much easier than beginning with a heavy racquet. Intermediate skills are easier to learn in racquetball than they are in either tennis or badminton as the shorter, lighter racquet handle enhances hand-eye-object coordination. Figure 3.1 shows examples of activities demanding good coordination.

POWER

Power is characterized by the explosiveness a force may produce. This eruptive power may be enhanced by improving both strength and speed. Strength can be improved some 50 percent through the use of isotonic or isometric exercises. Either or both of these techniques may be used, slightly increasing the workload to four or five days per week. Weightlifing is considered to be the quickest way to develop strength; however, considerable progress has been achieved through the use of calisthenics and mechanical devices such as the exer-genie, bicycle ergometer, treadmill and other pieces

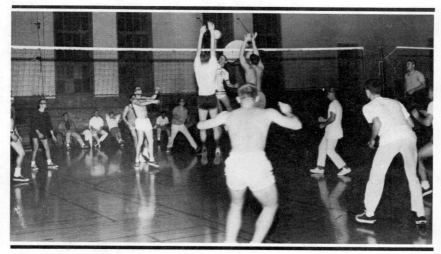

Figure 3.1c *Block that shot!*

of equipment designed for this purpose. Figure 3.2 shows examples of exercises you may use to develop power.

REACTION TIME

This term is used to define the interval of time required to respond to a stimulus. Fast reaction time is necessary for success in many sports. Speed of movement, ability to alter direction, and general body coordination are the fundamental ingredients and they can be improved by some 8 to 10 percent. The state of readiness, along with superior technical skills, seems to improve the reaction to a stimulus.

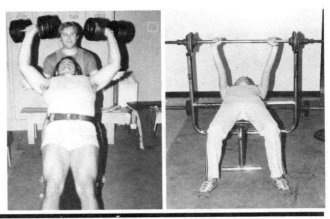

Figure 3.2a *Triceps lift* **Figure 3.2b** *Bench press*

If you don't have split-second response to numerous situational stimuli, you will be handicapped. Even though most of this quality appears to be hereditary, some gain may be realized through practicing specific movement patterns. The badminton smash is a good activity through which to work at improving reaction time. (See Figure 3.3.)

Figure 3.2c *Half-squat lift* **Figure 3.2d** *Bench press*

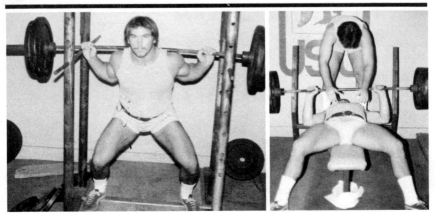

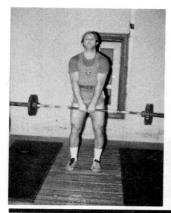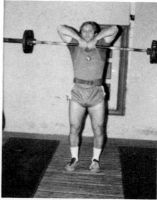

Figure 3.2e and f *Upright rowing exercise*

BODY MECHANICS

Good body mechanics implies the most efficient, effective, movement possible. It not only entails improving coordination, power, and reaction time, but learning how to use the body safely in all physical movements. In a broad sense, it is associated with recommended postural activities and includes the physical laws of movement.

Figure 3.3a *Ready position*   **Figure 3.3b** *Round-the-head smash*

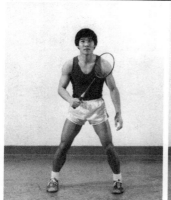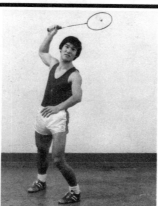

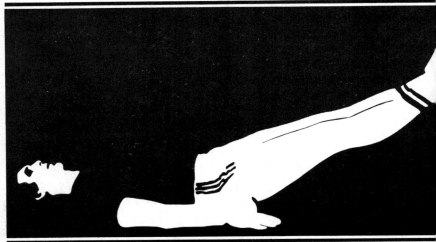

ASSESSMENT INVENTORY

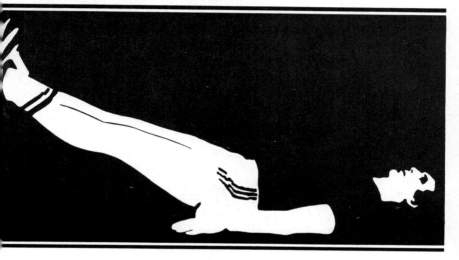

SYMMETRY AND POSTURE

Be concerned not only with how your body functions but also how it looks! Too many people have poor posture and ineffective body mechanics, and are asymmetrical. We immediately become concerned if our house sags, our furniture is misarranged, or our car is out of alignment, but give little attention to the development of a symmetrical body. It is as though we assume that nature will make the corrections or that the necessary alterations are impossible. In either case, nothing could be farther from the truth. The body functions more efficiently and looks better when there is a balance or harmonious arrangement of the body segments. It all depends on how important our appearance and physical condition is to us. Within reason, we can improve personal appearance, symmetrical development, and physical condition. Perhaps first we should answer the following questions: How does my appearance and physical condition compare with what I wish to be? How much of what I am at present would I like to retain? How much time and effort am I willing to commit for the achievement of the results?

Physical fitness, symmetrical development, and general appearance are very personal things. No one else can achieve them for us, and to acquire them requires a personal commitment. One thing we know—we can develop and maintain a high level of fitness, symmetrical contouring of the body, good posture, and effective body mechanics by participating in suitable developmental exercises.

Symmetry implies a correspondence of form and identity on opposite sides of a dividing line or axis. The left arm and leg should correspond in size and strength with the right arm and right leg. This applies to other bilateral parts of the body. The life style we have chosen tends to promote asymmetrical development. Many of the sports in which we participate fail to emphasize the uniform development of corresponding body segments. A right-handed tennis player should select a compatible exercise that would develop the left side. Some *cross development* takes place during exercise, but not enough to maintain a symmetrical configuration. Without a doubt, the congruent body functions more economically and efficiently than one lacking symmetrical development.

An inventory assessment check form has been included at the end of this chapter on which you may record your various fitness measurements. Repetition of these tests at regular intervals provides an opportunity to analyze the physiological changes that may result from your chosen life style. The value of recording the dates and measurement scores is that you can make comparisons of gains or losses. It is not necessary to have an exact measurement of physical fitness. However, it is important for everyone to have a relative assessment of his own fitness.

Posture refers to the characteristic way of bearing the body, especially the trunk and head. There is no universal posture that would be ideal for everyone. However, there are basic principles applicable to most body types. The way a person carries himself can be influential in minimizing the wear and tear on body segments due to use and the aging process. Some have suggested that faulty body carriage negatively influences one's personality, health, vitality and the impression one makes on others.

One should not attempt to correct any structural deviation, but functional deviations may be eradicated with appropriate exercise. Extensive use of a poorly aligned body may put a strain on the joints and surrounding tissues; unless this irregular posture is corrected, cumulative impairment is possible.

The use of a posture grid screen or plumb line is valuable in discovering anterior-posterior postural deviations. The following fundamental check points may also prove to be helpful in recognizing postural abnormalities. Authorities recommend that we:

1. Sit tall, with head and spine fully extended (Figure 4.1). Don't slump; place related bones end on end. Sit well back in a chair.

2. Stand tall, with head and spine fully extended (Figure 4.2). Use a plumb line test to assure vertical alignment. Gravity continuously challenges the anti-gravity muscles and tends to depress the trunk. We must forever guard against the unconscious development of *kyphosis* (hump back), *lordosis* (sway back), *scoliosis* (lateral curvature), or a combination of these deviations.

3. Walk tall. Move in a fully upright position, head high, chin in, shoulders back as though you own the world!

4. Guard against the development of:
   a) Forward head
   b) Tilted head
   c) Uneven shoulders (one shoulder slightly higher than the other)

d) Uneven hips (one hip slightly higher than the other)
e) Toes pointed out (they should be straight ahead)
f) Pronated or supinated ankles
g) Protuding abdomen
h) Weak arches

5. Lastly, guard against increased and decreased pelvic inclination, as either intensifies the exertion of the pelvic-lumbar relationship. Should this irregular inclination be permitted, it will be followed by chronic low back difficulties. A posture screen test (Figure 4.3) can help to discover irregularities of posture.

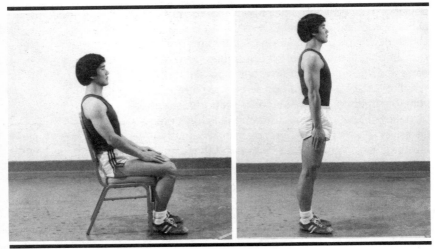

Figure 4.1 *Sit tall*   **Figure 4.2 *Stand tall***

PRECONDITIONING

Before beginning a strenuous physical conditioning program it is advisable to inaugurate a judicious preconditioning schedule. Many people neglect the value of preconditioning in preventing unnecessary soreness, and possible tissue injury. The length of time required, and the intensity of each workout, will depend upon a person's fitness level, interval of inactivity, and physiological age. If there has been a long period of inactivity, the preconditioning period should extend from three to six weeks. However, for most college-age people, two to three weeks should be adequate.

Basically, the preconditioning program should consist of big muscle activities such as walking, hiking, calisthenics, stretching, jogging, cycling, swimming, and so on. Space these activities throughout the day, never overdo at any one time. The total exercise time at the beginning should not exceed 45 to 60 minutes per day. As you become conditioned, you may increase the time and allot larger chunks of time to the specific activities you want to include in your exercise program.

Discernible soreness resulting from workouts is usually indicative of overexertion. Overtaxing of unconditioned tissues must be avoided. However, each

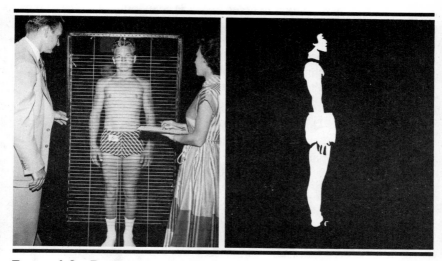

Figure 4.3 *Posture screen test*

workout should be incrementally intensified unless the symptoms of negative effects have been observed.

Warmup.

This is a term that refers to the preparatory phase of an exercise bout, or athletic event. It includes calisthenics, which seem to enhance the diffusion of gases in the cardiorespiratory system, and the stretching of specific reciprocal muscle groups and connective tissues. The warmup should enhance the strength, accuracy and range of selected movement patterns. Athletes and coaches believe that the warmup will prevent a significant number of athletic injuries.

FLEXIBILITY

Flexibility is a term used to describe the range of motion by various body segments. In many parts of the body, movement is limited by bony structure, type of joint, bulk of related muscles, and the degree to which tissues can be stretched. The newborn baby is usually very flexible. But as the child ages, there seems to be a shortening of the connective tissue that surrounds joints. This is usually due to disuse or misuse, which may result in debilitative injury. Inadequate flexibility usually affects both aesthetic and efficient movement potential.

Dynamic flexibility contributes to graceful, effective, movement patterns, and is considered to help in the prevention of tissue injury. Precaution is essential in the use of both static and ballistic stretching in order to avoid muscle or tendon injury. Therefore, you should gradually increase your flexibility over a long period of time. The techniques which follow have proved satisfactory in the stretching of various muscle groups.

1) Bend and Stretch (hamstrings)

Starting position: Standing, feet some 18 inches apart.

1. With knees slightly flexed, touch fingers to the floor.
2. Slowly return to starting position.
3. Repeat for one minute.

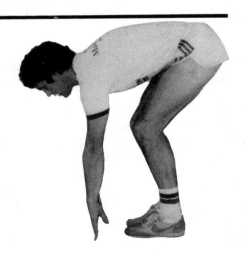

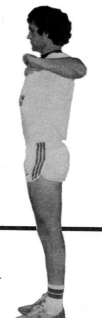

2) **Wing Stretch (chest)**
Starting position: Standing, feet slightly apart, upper arm parallel to floor, fist clenched in front of chest.
1. Thrust elbows backward.
2. Return to starting position.
3. Repeat for one minute.

3) **Body Bender (lower back)**
Starting position: Standing, fingers interlaced behind neck.
1. Bend sideward to the right.
2. Return to starting position.
3. Bend sidward to the left.
4. Return to starting position.
5. Repeat for one minute.

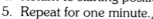

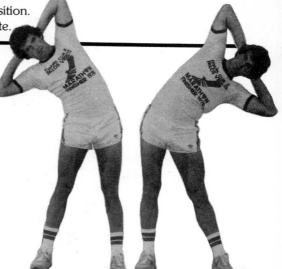

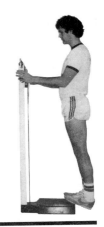

4) Ankle Stretch (calf extension)
Starting position: Stand with balls of feet on object, arms extended forward.

1. Lower heels.
2. Return to starting position.
3. Raise heels.
4. Return to starting position.
5. Repeat several times.

5) Sitting Stretch (trunk flexion)
Starting position: Sitting on floor, back straight, hands on knees.

1. Bend forward, extending hands as far as possible.
2. Return to starting position.
3. Repeat several times.

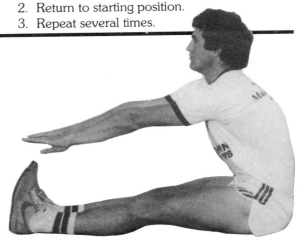

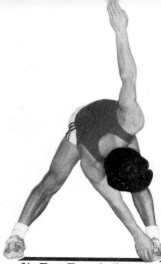

6) Toe Touch (hamstring, low back, rotator muscles)

Starting position: Standing, feet shoulder width apart, arms extended upward.

1. Bend downward, touch fingers outside right foot.
2. Return to starting position.
3. Bend downward, touch fingers outside left foot.
4. Return to starting position.
5. Repeat several times.

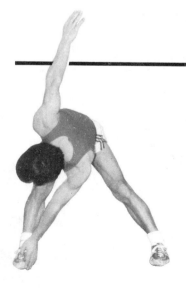

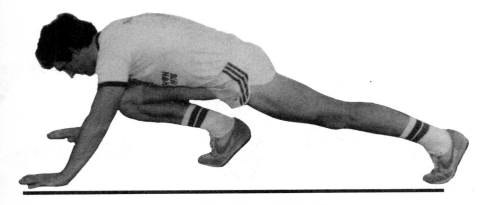

7) Knee-to-Head Stretch (back)

Starting position: On all fours.

1. Right knee toward head.
2. Return to starting position.
3. Left knee toward head.
4. Return to starting position.
5. Repeat several times.

8) Achilles Stretch (Achilles tendon)

Starting position: Stand arm's length from wall.

1. Place hands on wall, body straight, touch head to wall, person or other resistant object.
2. Return to starting position.
3. Repeat several times.

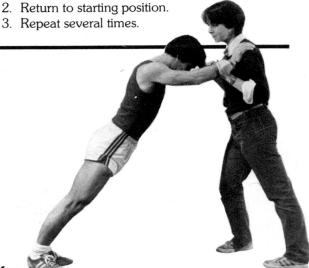

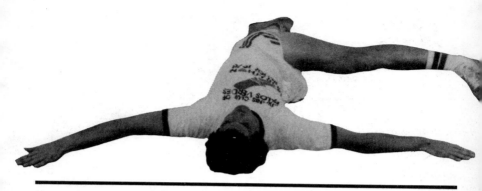

9) Leg Over (trunk rotators)

Starting position: Lie on back, arms extended
sidewards.

1. Bring straight left leg across body until left toe
   touches extended right hand.
2. Return to starting position.
3. Bring straight right leg across body until right
   toe touches left hand.
4. Return to starting position.
5. Repeat several times.

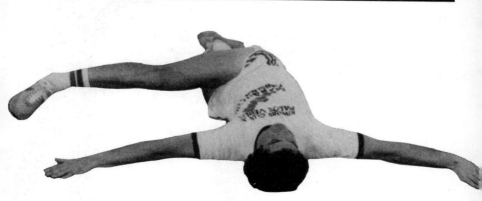

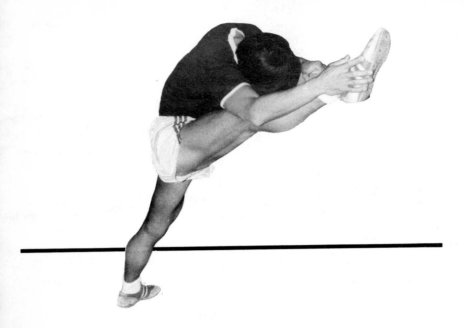

10) Bench Stretch (hamstrings)

Starting position: Stand, left leg extended on table, right foot on floor.

1. Keep right foot on floor, bend forward and touch beyond toes.
2. Return to starting position.
3. Repeat several times.
4. Reverse position and repeat exercise, stretching other side of body.

11) Sitting Curl (back extensors)

Starting position: Sit on bench, back straight, hands on knees, feet flat on floor.

1. Tuck, extend hands between legs under bench as far backward as possible.
2. Return to starting position.
3. Repeat several times.

(The monkey roll, demonstrated in the next exercise, is another back extensor exercise.)

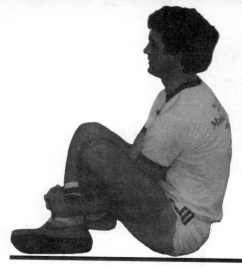

12) Monkey Roll (rotatory muscles)

Starting position: Sit on floor, hands extended inside knees, over the legs and fingers clasped.

1. Keeping hands clasped, roll in a circle, first one way then the other.
2. Repeat several times.

13) Back Rocker (spine stretcher)

Starting position: Sit on floor, knees drawn to chest, hands clasped below knees.

1. Rock backwards on to upper back.
2. Rock to starting position.
2. Repeat several times.

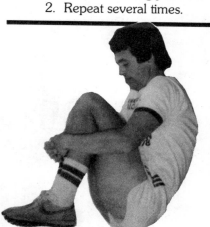 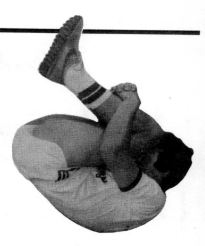

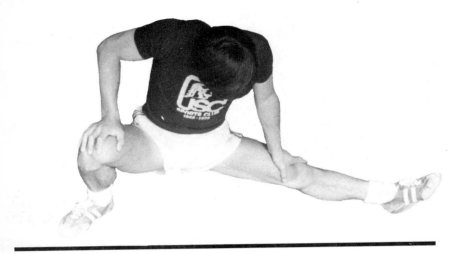

---

14) Stride Stretcher (back and leg)

Starting position: On hands and feet.

1. Jump slightly, bring right knee as far forward as possible, simultaneously extend left leg backward.
2. Push hips toward floor.
3. Return to starting position.
4. Reverse the action: left knee forward, right leg extended. Push hips toward floor.
5. Return to starting position.
6. Repeat several times.

Exercise 15

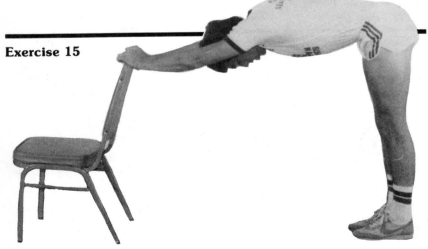

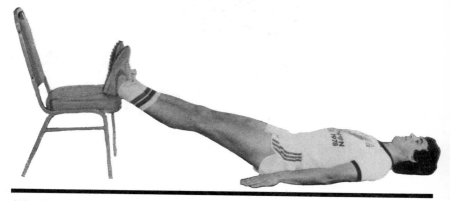

15) Chair Stretcher (chest-pectorals)

Starting position: Stand facing back of chair; bend forward, place hands on back of chair.

1. Keep back straight, draw head and chest downward.
2. Return to starting position.
3. Repeat several times.

16) Elevated Curl-ups (abdomen)

Starting position: Lie on floor, face up, heels elevated on chair, arms at side.

1. Slowly curl forward, touch hands to toes.
2. Return slowly to starting position.
3. Repeat several times.

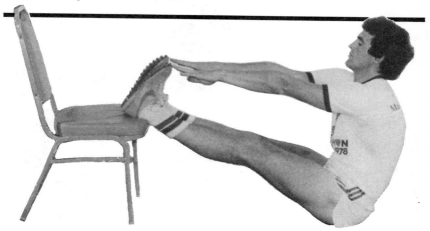

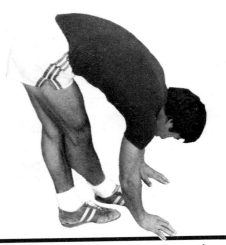

17) Pull Stretcher (back, hamstrings, gluteus)

Starting position: Sit facing partner, legs spread at a 45° angle, feet in contact; grasp partner's hands.

1. Pull partner as far forward as possible.
2. Reverse the pull.
3. Repeat several times.

You may prefer the exercise shown above.

18) Bend and Reach (back, gluteus, hamstrings)

Starting position: Stand on a bench.

1. Keep legs straight, bend from waist; measure how far from the floor in front of toes the fingers are. (Measure in inches.)
2. Return to starting position.
3. Repeat several times.

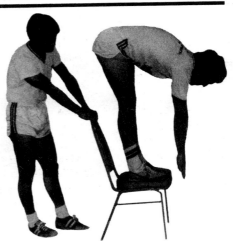

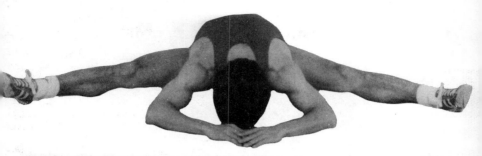

19) Sit and Reach (back and hamstrings)

Starting position: Sit on floor, legs straight, feet against an immovable object.

1. Extend arms, flex body, reach as far beyond object as possible. Measure reach in inches.
2. Return to starting position.
3. Repeat several times.

Or you may prefer the exercise shown in the photograph.

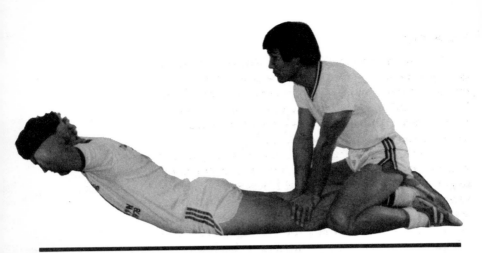

20) Trunk Extension (trunk extensors and flexors)

Starting position: Lie face down, fingers interlocked behind head, partner holding buttock and legs down. This exercise may also be done without a partner, as shown below.

1. Raise head and shoulders as high as possible. Measure distance from floor to nose in inches.
2. Relax to starting position.
3. Repeat several times.

Additional activities that may be used to enhance flexibility are:

1) Hanging from a bar, rings, tree limbs, etc.
2) Floating on water.
3) Hanging from an object with the legs.

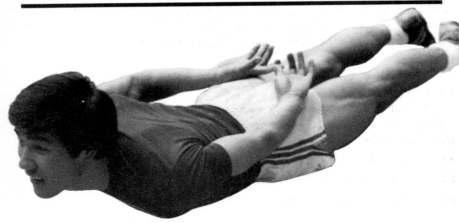

ENDURANCE

It is strongly recommended that a three to six week general conditioning period precede any intensive endurance training. This is particularly important if you have been living a sedentary life or recovering from a recent illness. If there is any question about cardiac insufficiency, consult your physician.

After using the overload principle in a daily graduated exercise program for three to six weeks, you should be ready to determine your physical fitness level. Take the various field tests listed in this chapter. Enter the date and scores on the physical fitness profile form at the end of the chapter. By systematic testing and recording of the data, the longitudinal story of your fitness may be observed. Occasional analysis of the data will reveal whether you are losing or gaining in physical efficiency.

Exercise programs should be on a regular basis, never less than three times a week; testing should always be under similar conditions such as the same time of day, the same distance from the last meal, etc.

The longitudinal records of the fitness profile may reveal physiological changes helpful in the maintenance of health. A sedentary life style, together with increasing age, will necessitate additional exercise for fitness retention.

Keep in mind that the three to six week preconditioning period should include some 60 minutes of exercise daily—not necessarily vigorous nor all at the same time. *And*, it should include three to four 30 minute weekly bouts of sustained activity such as jogging, basketball, dancing, cycling, or fast walking.

The following activities are suggested as measures of endurance.

The Step Test. A very reliable heart-rate recovery test can be measured as follows:

Step up and down on a 16 to 18 inch high bench for a three to five minute period at a cadence of 25 to 30 steps per minute.

a) Record resting heart rate *prior* to the step test.

b) Take the step test.

c) Record your recovery rate:

1 – 1½ minutes after the step test _____

2 – 2½ minutes after the step test _____

3 – 3½ minutes after the step test _____

Your cardiovascular recovery index relates to the sum of the three 30 second counts. It has been estimated that if they total

        95 – 120—Take a deep bow you are super!

        121 – 135—Better than most people

        136 – 150—A little above average

        151 – 165—Just average

        166 – 180—There's a problem ahead

        181 – 200—There are problems now!

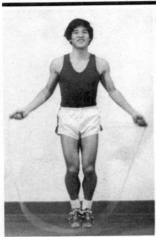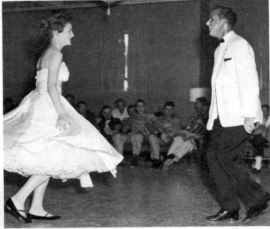

Figure 4.4 *Rope skipping*

Figure 4.5 *A good fast square dance will build endurance . . .*

After completing the test, record the scores on your profile form.

    If for some reason you do not wish to use the step test to measure your cardiovascular recovery rate, one of the following activities may be used for the same purpose. Use the same measurements for the step test, and record the data for future comparison.

a) Rope skipping (Figure 4.4)

b) Bicycle riding (uphill or speed racing)

c) Dancing—polka, samba, tap, disco, square (Figure 4.5) and folk (Figure 4.6)

d) Wood chopping

e) Running in place

f) Jogging for five minutes

Two-Mile Run. One of the most reliable field tests for measuring aerobic capacity is the two-mile run. However, only preconditioned individuals should attempt this strenuous test.

The following listed times for this distance present a reliable estimate of cardiorespiratory fitness.

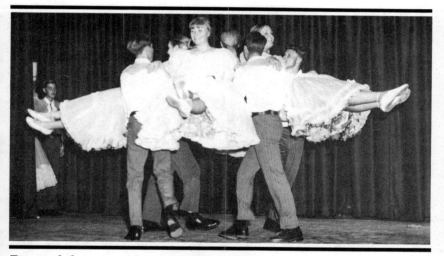

Figure 4.6 *. . . and so will the swing*

10 – 12 minutes—Take a deep bow—you are super!
12 – 13 minutes—Better than most
13 – 14 minutes—Above average
14 – 15 minutes—Average
15 – 17 minutes—Problems ahead
17+ minutes—You have problems now!

All that is required is preconditioning for at least three weeks, a watch, and marked-off distance.

If you do not want your cardiorespiratory system to age prematurely, start a regular exercise program now. It should become a part of your life style. Jog, run, work, play games, do calisthenics, be active—it's a major way to slow down the aging process.

STRENGTH

Strength is the physical capability of generating a sustained reaction to resist force, attack, strain or stress. Without considerable strength you will tire easily, miss numerous adventures, become a slave to modern conveniences, and make a poor recovery from sickness and accidents, thus missing more work than necessary.

Strength and endurance can be improved by utilization of the overload principle. That is, gradually increase the work load. For instance, if ten chin-ups are

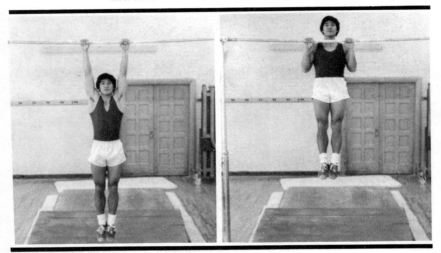

Figure 4.7

difficult today, try eleven the next day, and so on until the desired fitness of the biceps and other related muscles has been realized. This same procedure may be used by selecting appropriate exercises for all muscle groups.

The following activities are suggested to measure and develop strength.

Chinups. Chin-ups are used to develop strength in the biceps and other arm and shoulder muscles (Figure 4.7). The procedure for doing this simple exercise follows.

a) **Equipment:** Overhead bar slightly higher than your grasp when standing beneath it; or other modified equipment such as a tree limb, door-jamb bar, rings, etc.

b) **Starting position:** jump and grasp bar, palms forward, about shoulder width apart.

c) From a fully extended position pull the body upwards until the chin is slightly above the bar.

d) Slowly return to the extended position.

e) Repeat (add a count each time the chin clears the bar).

The strength of the arm and shoulder muscles may be estimated by the number of chin-ups you can do.

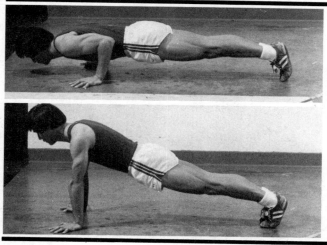

Figure 4.8

> 20+ —Take a bow—you are super!
> 17 – 20—Better than most
> 13 – 16—Better than average
> 9 – 11—M—m—m kind of average
> 6 – 8—Problems ahead
> Below 6—Problems now!

Push-ups. Push-ups are used to strengthen the abdominal muscles as well as those in the arm and shoulder (Figure 4.8). The procedure for doing this exercise is as follows:

a) **Starting position:** Lie on floor face down, legs extended, hands shoulder width apart, weight supported by hands and toes. (If difficult, use modified procedure with knees on floor instead of toes.)

b) Keep the body straight and push full arm length away from the floor.

c) Return to starting position but only touch chin to floor.

d) Repeat and keep a running count of push-ups.

The strength of your muscles may be estimated by the number of push-ups you can do.

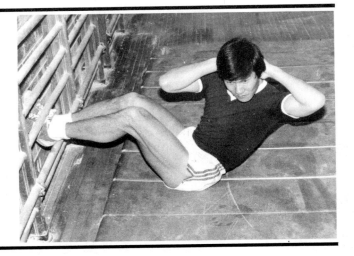

Figure 4.9

30+ —Hi, champ, you are very good!
25 – 30—Better than most
15 – 25—Better than average
12 – 14—M—m—m about average
8 – 11—Problems ahead
Below 8—Problems now!

Take the test, record date and score, see if you can improve.

Bent Knee Sit-Ups. These are used to strengthen the abdominal muscles (Figure 4.9).

a) Starting position: Lie on back, hands behind head, knees bent, feet tucked between wall bars, or under a heavy object such as a chest or bed.

b) Raise upper body to a sitting position, elbows touching knees.

c) Return to starting position.

d) Repeat, keep count. (Mark scores after exercise is over.)

The strength of the abdominal muscles may be estimated by the number of sit-ups you can perform:

PHYSICAL FITNESS PROFILE (Self testing—Easy to do—See how you change)							
Date							
Height							
Weight							
ENDURANCE: Step Test Score							
Rope Skipping							
Two Mile Run							
STRENGTH: Number Chin-ups							
Number Push-ups							
Number Sit-ups							
FLEXIBILITY: Bend and Reach							
Sit and Reach							
HOURS YOU EXERCISE PER WEEK							

30+ —Marvelous!
24 – 29—Better than most
17 – 23—Above average
12 – 16—Uh! About average
8 – 11—Problems ahead
Below 8—Problems now!

5

NUTRITION, EXERCISE AND WEIGHT CONTROL

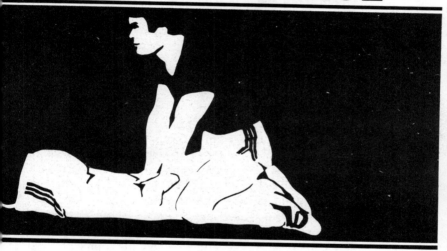

We eat too much! It is a bad American custom. Furthermore, we eat too much of the wrong kind of food. Often this is due to the bad habits, attitudes and patterns developed during childhood. A major weakness is that we become addicted to certain foods with a high caloric value.

A *calorie* is the quantity of heat required to raise the temperature of one gram of water by 1°C from a standard initial temperature at one atmospheric pressure. The caloric value of a specific food is determined by dehydrating the food and burning it in a special container, called a *calorimeter*. There are approximately 4.0 calories per gram in carbohydrates and in proteins. But fats contain approximately 9.0 calories per gram. To maintain weight, the intake of calories should not exceed the number used in a day's activity.

The *basal metabolic rate* is the number of calories required per day when one is at complete rest. Basal metabolic rate can be estimated by multiplying body weight (in pounds) by eleven. A person at rest who weighs 150 pounds requires 1,650 calories per day to maintain his weight.

People involved in vigorous work or play may require 5,000 – 6,000 calories per day. As weight increases, there is a proportional increase in metabolism, both at rest and at play. Furthermore, weight gain and weight loss are proportional to calorie intake and to calorie expenditure. The thyroid gland secretes a hormone, thyroxin, which helps to regulate the metabolic rate.

FOODS

The body's basic nutrients may be divided into five categories—proteins, carbohydrates, fats, vitamins, and minerals.

Proteins are a group of complex nitrogenous organic compounds of high molecular weight that contain amino acids as their basic structural unit. Protein is a substance found in all living matter and essential for the growth and repair of animal tissue. It is the main content of the body and is present in all tissues. There are about 25 sub-units in a protein molecule called amino acids. Meat, fish, poultry, milk, cheese, and bread are the source of protein. Since protein calories are not readily stored in the body, the quantity consumed is not likely to unduly affect weight. Their major function is to build, repair, and regulate cell function. The word protein is derived from a Greek word meaning "holding first place."

Increased protein intake is recommended if the objective is to build lean muscle mass, but most authorities agree that high protein pre-game meals are of minimum value.

Carbohydrates supply energy for work and play. They are composed of chemical compounds, including sugars, starches, and cellulose containing carbon, hydrogen, and oxygen. The most familiar sugars are glucose (found in fruits and honey), fructose (found in fruit), sucrose (found in sugar cane, sugar beets and fruit), lactose (from milk), and maltase (found in malt). Starches are found in cereal grains and in potatoes. Sugars are converted into glycogen (blood sugar) and readily stored in the liver and in the muscle tissues. If the intake is excessive it is converted into fat, which may lead to obesity. Some glycogen is continually carried in the blood where it is immediately available and necessary for muscular contractions.

Fats are any of various soft solid or semisolid organic compounds comprising the glyceride esters of fatty acids and other related compounds. They are a secondary source of energy and may be found in butter, margarine, oils, meats, whole milk, chocolate and in all kinds of nuts. Fats are a more concentrated form of fuel than carbohydrates and proteins.

Minerals are as essential as proteins, carbohydrates and fats. They act in conjunction with vitamins, and without one the other is useless. A few of the minerals are so essential they should be a part of your daily diet. Those considered most important are listed on a chart at the end of the chapter.

Vitamins are chemical substances found in both animal and vegetable matter. They promote normal growth, maintain health, and prevent and/or cure certain diseases. An adequate daily supply may be obtained from a good variety of basic foods.

Malnutrition.

Far too many people are unaware of the life-taking diseases brought on by hunger and malnutrition. These diseases may not be as dramatic as heart failure or cancer, but they are just as deadly and just as unpleasant to talk about. The problem is greater in some other parts of the world than it is in the United States, since we live in the world's bread basket. Nevertheless, there is considerable malnutrition in this country. Some of it is due to ignorance, some to greediness, some to shiftlessness, and some to poverty. In far too many poor homes there is less nutritious food on the table than there is in the garbage pails of the rich. The health and nutritional care of the poor, the old, the very young, and the unfortunate, is a national disgrace. It's a challenge for all of us to do what we can about it.

Obesity.

Overweight is usually due to consuming more calories than are used. It's just that simple. Everyone should watch his diet, exercise regularly, get enough sleep, practice good hygiene and avoid excesses.

There are a number of ways you can measure to find out if you are getting fat. Everyone can use one of the following methods.

1. Honest visual appraisal. Examine yourself in the mirror!

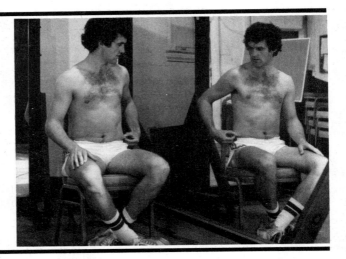

Figure 5.1 *Pinch test above hip*

2. Skinfold or pinch test. If you do not have a caliper for measurement, a pinch test will serve just as well. The objective is to find out the amount of fat that *exists* beneath the skin and over the muscles. If more than one-half inch separates the thumb and forefinger in one or more places, you're getting fat! Measurements should be made in four places, just above the hip in line with armpit (Figure 5.1), the middle of the triceps (Figure 5.2), midway on the biceps, and just below the shoulder blade.

3. Body composition or body density measurement. The most accurate measurement of body composition is the underwater weighing technique. However, this method is not practical for most individuals. This measurement is based on the principle that residual air volume can be estimated and gross underwater weight determined. Since the density of bone and muscle tissue is heavier than water, and of fatty tissue less than water, a fairly accurate body composition measurement may be ascertained. Pollock, Wilmore and Fox have described rather precisely the underwater measurement technique in their book *Health and Fitness Through Physical Activity.*

Recommended body fat composition for college age men and women is as follows:

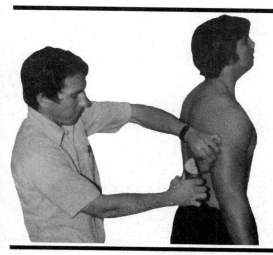

Figure 5.2 *Skinfold test on triceps with calipers*

Body Fat	Men	Women
Below average	6 – 12%	9 – 15%
Average	12 – 15%	16 – 20%
Above average	16+	21+

EXERCISE AND WEIGHT CONTROL

The basic structural unit of the body is the cell. Every part of the body is composed of millions of tiny cells. There are skin cells, muscle cells, blood cells, nerve cells, and bone cells. Each varies in size and shape depending on location and function. Furthermore, each cell has the ability to reproduce itself.

THE BODY'S VITAMIN AND MINERAL NEEDS

Name	Source	Function in the Body	Servings Daily
Vitamin A	Butter, cheese, cod liver oil, egg yolk, leafy green vegetables, liver, yellow vegetables, and tomatoes	Promotes normal vision and growth; maintains general health	One
Vitamin B Complex	Lean pork, liver, egg yolk, whole grains, beans, peas, nuts, fruits, vegetables	Stimulates appetite; aids digestion; promotes growth; regulates nervous system	Two
Vitamin C	Citrus fruits, other fresh fruits, berries, cabbage, greens, fresh vegetables, sprouted legumes	Maintains connective tissue; assists in the development of bones and teeth; aids cell activity; strengthens blood vessels and body tissues	Two (cannot be stored)
Vitamin D	Eggs, liver, fish, sunshine	Essential for bone and teeth development, promotes growth	One
Vitamin E	Egg yolk, cereals, lettuce, spinach, corn oil	Promotes general well-being, mental and physical vigor, good muscle tone	One
Calcium	Almonds, cheese, dry beans, egg yolk, milk, leafy vegetables, molasses	Assists in the development of bones and teeth; aids blood clotting; essential for healthy muscles and nerves	Two
Copper	Avocadoes, dry beans, peas, liver, oats, corn, whole wheat	Aids cell activity; prevents certain anemias	One
Iodine	Seafoods, fish, foods grown near the ocean, iodized salt	Encourages normal growth; prevents goiter	One
Iron	Berries, fruits, dried fruits, dried beans, peas, eggs, lean meats, bread, green vegetables, molasses, rye flour, whole wheat, oatmeal	Builds hemoglobin and other carriers of oxygen; prevents some anemias	One
Phosphorus	Cheese, dried beans, liver, nuts, flour	Stimulates and aids cell activity; assists in the development of bones and teeth	One
Potassium	Dried apricots, dates, figs, dried beans, molasses, nuts, soy flour	Promotes growth; stimulates and aids cell activity; essential for healthy heart, nerves and muscles	One
Sodium	Bread, butter, cheese, salmon, table salt	Helps maintain water balance; prevents fatigue	One

Similar cells are grouped together to form the body's tissues. Two or more tissues grouped together to perform certain functions (such as the heart, lungs, brain, eyes, liver, kidneys, stomach and intestines), are called organs. A system is an arrangement of organs concerned with the same function.

The health of all cells, tissues, organs, and systems depends upon good nutrition, adequate rest, appropriate exercise, freedom from disease and efficient movement patterns. Highly effective and efficient movement patterns are rarely developed except by a few extraordinary persons. Those who do master efficient movement patterns can maintain them through most of their life with minimal debilitating effects from wear and tear. However, excessive and inefficient neuromuscular patterns, along with accidental injuries, may bring an early onset of limited movement, resulting in the forceful termination of an athlete's career long before he has peaked.

The human skeleton, like any machine, works more efficiently when in balance. Body deviations are quite common, sometimes due to illness, injury, malnutrition, lack of development, or genetic effects. Most deviations are the result of improper movement patterns maintained since early childhood. The point is, you should be aware of any body deviation you have, and make sure the exercise you select improves rather than harms your posture.

The body burns nutrients just as a power plant burns fuel. It is essential that you always maintain a proper nutrient level, otherwise the body system lacks the ingredients needed to develop adequately.

Exercised muscle cells tend to enlarge. This compensatory growth is referred to as *hypertrophy*. Concomitantly, exercise requires the burning of calories. The more vigorously and routinely you exercise, the more you are able to use excessive intake of calories. Authorities agree that exercise, not diet, is the easiest and most predictable way to lose or maintain weight. It is possible for an individual to preserve the desired weight by maintaining a balance between food intake and calorie expenditure.

In certain vigorous activities such as climbing, running, rowing, and wrestling as many as 700 calories per hour can be used. Vigorous participation in badminton, basketball, bicycling, dancing, gymnastics, handball, hill climbing, jogging, skating, skiing, soccer, squash, swimming, tennis, and volleyball requires some 500 to 600 calories per hours. Participation in the above activities in a more moderate manner is likely to burn some 400 to 500 calories per hour.

To be successful in using exercise to help achieve weight control, you must select carefully the type and quantity of movement necessary. The best way to maintain weight control is to regulate calorie intake with

calorie expenditure. If you depend on diet alone you will probably be constantly hungry. Exercise just prior to mealtime helps curb the appetite. But when trying to reduce, never attempt to lose more that two pounds per week.

Those who have made a scientific study of the human body recognize that it is designed for action. In other words, the body functions best when used regularly. Furthermore, unless abused, it is nearly impossible to wear it out. The human body, when used properly, has tremendous resilience. Modern industrialization and automation have greatly reduced physical demands on the body that were once part of

earning a living. This reduction in work-energy
expenditure has made it necessary to supplement the
modern life style with exercise programs. To keep weight
at a respectable level, calorie intake must be balanced
with energy output; it's that simple. So select activities
that burn up those extra calories. It can add zest to your
life. And keep in mind that increasing your activity is more
important that decreasing your food intake.

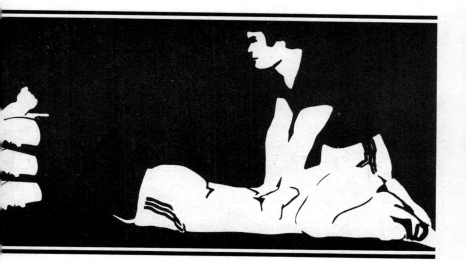

6

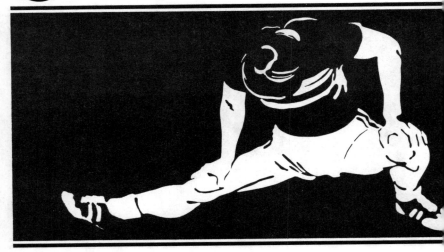

LEARNING PHYSICAL SKILLS

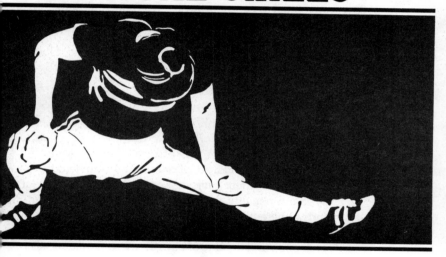

Participation in various sports may be used in lieu of calisthenics, weight lifting, or jogging for the development and maintenance of physical fitness. If this is your choice, it is to your advantage to develop at least middle-range proficiency in your preferred sports. Working to learn and improve physical skills may enhance your entire life style, because it seems that the better skilled are more active than those with less proficiency. An excellent way to maintain high-level fitness is to be active. Therefore, one's movement skills should be as advanced as possible.

Skill learning can be defined as a gain in knowledge,

comprehension, and improvement in or about a motor movement. In a sense, it implies an improvement in the performance of a preferred motor movement. If the change in proficiency is to be classified as learned it cannot be the result of an organismic variable such as maturity.

TYPES OF LEARNING

Most authorities tend to group the acquisition of knowledge and abilities into one of three categories; affective, cognitive, and effective learning.

Affective learning implies an attitudinal change. Cognitive learning relates to mental processes and is conceptual in nature. Effective learning implies that there is a change in movement skills. Both cognitive and effective learning take place during the acquisition of new skills. Movement patterns must be remembered if they are to be consciously repeated.

HEREDITY

How we look, think, and move is strongly influenced by our heredity. This term is often defined as the totality of characteristics, traits, and associated potentialities transmitted to an individual organism. Basic heredity includes the genetic traits fused together at the moment the sperm penetrates the ova. But there are two other kinds of heredity that also influence us in many ways.

During the nine months between the moment of conception and the day of birth, numerous influences are transmitted to the unborn fetus, and these make up *congenital heredity*. During this period of time, it is extremely important that the mother maintains good health and enjoys a nutritious diet. Otherwise, the fetus may receive negative influences that result in permanent damage.

The term *environmental heredity* is used to describe the pragmatic influences that affect a person's development. We observe people, we copy their movements which then become part of us. Sometimes this is an advantage; sometimes not. Too frequently we fail to discriminate in the selection of movements to imitate. This is especially true of motor skills. Most individual movements are spontaneous and analytically unrehearsed. Early in life we begin to develop a host of erroneous and uncomplimentary movements, and few people are knowledgeable enough to tell us a better way to run, throw, or hit an object.

Different combinations of hereditary traits and influences produce people who differ from one another. Not only are your abilities different from those of other people, but so are your likes, dislikes, and aspirations, shaped by a multitude of germinating influences.

Heredity includes the accumulation of traits and influences that an individual receives from genetic, congenital or environmental sources. Collectively, these traits are influential in determining an individual's total configuration. Furthermore, these characteristics are extremely influential in structuring an individual's life style and fitness. An analysis of someone's heredity will often reveal the cause that inhibits his ability to learn.

LEARNING MOTOR SKILLS

We begin to learn gross motor movements while still in the womb. After birth, we learn how to lift our head, reach for objects, sit, stand and resist gravity as we walk. Slowly but progressively we learn to feed ourselves, talk, and initiate those movements that are characteristic in the mature adult. Thousands of trials precede every refined movement. But those high-level skill movements essential for most sports seem to be more than most of us possess.

Why do so many adults have so much trouble playing a skillful game of tennis, golf, or any other sport? Most likely it is because we were never taught the skill correctly, and never developed the ability to analyze the necessary fundamental movements. The sequence by which motor skills are learned follows a rather definite pattern. In some instances it may require a substantial time span; there are people who have been playing golf for years and who still cannot make a straight shot.

First there is a pre-skill stage. This is the time when general physical conditioning occurs, gross movements are generalized and some conceptual ideas are formalized about the desired routine.

The second phase involves further conditioning along with practice of the whole desired routine.

This is followed by a third stage in which the whole routine is broken down into parts or sub-routines. The refinement of each sub-routine may require extensive practice. At this time a careful analysis should be made of related mechanical principles involved in each movement. Consideration should be given to utilizing a summation of forces whereby each muscle group is triggered to contract in a precise sequential order. In the execution of every correct routine there is a hierarchy of sub-routine movements.

As an example of proper sequencing, let us use the golf swing. In the book on golf in this series, Hardy and Walsh have emphasized that the golf swing is composed of five basic elements. They are the grip, stance, backswing, downswing, and follow-through. Each element needs to be individually analyzed, practiced, assembled in a sequential order and executed in a smooth fluid manner. Several different muscle groups are involved in the golf swing, and it is most important that each muscle group contracts in the proper order.

The fourth and final stage in which motor skills are learned is generally referred to as the maintenance stage. The practice of specialized routines and sub-routines requires persistence. For instance, skill in using the short irons in golf, with infrequent practice, seems to decline more rapidly than it does with woods. Some very good golfers have indicated that they must habitually practice their chip shots in order to retain their handicaps. These same considerations are factors in the maintenance of skills in most special activities. Find out which sub-routines require the most frequent practice. If this advice is followed a skill once learned is not difficult to retain.

LEARNING VARIABLES

An analysis of the following factors should speed up the time required to acquire skills, and will probably assist in their retention.

1. *Practice.* Most authorities agree that the practice of physical skills is more fruitful when it is done with a purpose. Many kinds of movement are beneficial in

the maintenance of fitness, but detailed practice on specific movements is essential for skill improvement. The length and frequency of practice sessions varies with the age and skill level of the participant, and strenuousness of the skill. (In the earlier stages of skill learning, rest periods should be included in the practice session.)

2. *Feedback.* Cue recognition that movements are done correctly is invaluable in shortening the learning process. Efforts should be made to duplicate superior movements. This seems to be far more valuable than trying to analyze an incorrect motion. Both auditory and visual cues are helpful. For example, an analysis of a golf ball in flight discloses the club head position at the point of impact. The "swish" sound of a badminton racquet reveals its velocity at the time of a smash. A smooth, accelerated striking motion is used in both the racquet sport and golf. The "ping" of a tennis ball hitting the "sweet spot" on the racquet indicates the accuracy of contact, and the dull sound of the shuttlecock striking wood is indicative of improper contact.

   Tactile perception by the cutaneous receptors provides useful information for the cerebral cortex, which in turn makes an initiatory decision regarding the improvement of a skill movement. However, unless the performer aspires to improve, the feedback may be useless.

   Detailed observation of a playing field; the problems that skiers are having with the terrain; the direction the wind is blowing; the position of the sun; the weakness an opponent has in executing specific skills; all are visual cues. Highly skilled performers make maximum use of this kind of information. Knowing about the spin or roll of a ball will help them anticipate its direction.

3. *Chunking.* It is sometimes easier to remember the sequence of several sub-routines by combining them into a larger category. As an example, two or three different dance steps may be sequentially grouped for memory retention.

4. *Muscle spindle reflex.* The greater the muscle stretch, the more forceful will be its contraction. However, if accuracy is also a factor, as in the golf swing, less stretch is usually advisable.

5. *Follow-through.* Usually a movement can be improved by extending it beyond the impact stage. An example is the follow-through when hitting a golf ball. This procedure tends to maximize the force used in hitting an object, and subsequently reduces the strain on the muscles involved in the movement.

6. *Reflex training.* Repetitive movements tend to develop a muscular reaction requiring minimal contraction. Examples are the blocking of a punch by a boxer, blocking a smash in badminton, avoiding a wild pitch in baseball. Star athletes display phenomenal reflex action.

7. *State of readiness.* Learning the most expedient position for both offensive and defensive attack is most advantageous. With the weight forward on both feet in a well-balanced, slightly crouched position, it is possible to move more quickly.

8. *Trial and success.* Successful competition is based upon hours of specific skill practice. At first, the experience may be classified as trial and error, but when the right movement has been mastered it is more rightfully called trial and success.

9. *Kinematics.* This is the science of motion. Students committed to improving their physical skills should study Sir Isaac Newton's laws of motion, which relate to acceleration, efficiency, motion, speed, torque, velocity, and work.

10. *Stress syndrome.* The physiological changes that occur during stressful situations such as exercise and disease do not seem to be different from those experienced in anger, fear or other social stress situations. Special attention should be given to over-heating, ventilation, proper amount of liquids, perspiration, and the kind of clothing worn when exercising in order to reduce stressful situations. A semi-relaxed performer experiences less stress.

11. *Overlearning.* The retention of skills is more likely when the movements are overlearned. That is, continue the practice drills even after the movement has been perfected.

12. *Ideakinesis.* Imagined movements are beneficial and frequently reduce the number of rehearsals that the learning of a specific movement requires. Mental imagery and mental practice are parts of every skillful performer's style. You see the flight of the ball before you execute the swing.

13. *Breath holding.* There is a mechanical advantage in holding your breath when executing specific movements such as a free throw in basketball, a

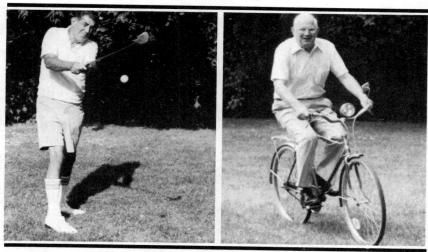

Figure 6.1a *Practicing the golf swing*
Figure 6.1b *A leisurely bike ride*

swing at a baseball, a golf swing, or a 100-yard dash. This is because fewer movements have to be coordinated.

14. *Transfer of learning.* Performers seem to believe that there is a greater transfer of learning in physical skills than researchers have been able to prove. However, specific practice on a selected movement seems to provide the greatest invariable improvement.

15. *Relaxed movement.* Skilled performers have found that it is less fatiguing when they perform in a relaxed manner.

THE JOY OF EFFORT

There is phenomenological pleasantness about being in motion. Just what occurs is uncertain. We think that it is a combination of numerous physiological, sociological and psychological variables. It is doubtful whether those who have never experienced this sensation really understand what we are taking about, and what they are missing. But, it's there anyway. Just ask active people why they are so movement oriented. The predominant

answer seems to be, "I feel better when I am active." (See Figure 6.1.) And it appears that the greatest joy is derived from substantial effort. This is also a little understood phenomenon. But it is a reality, and if you have not experienced this sensation, give it a try!

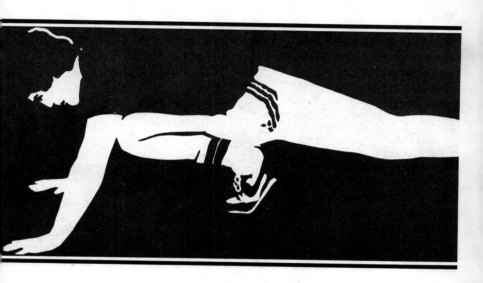

7

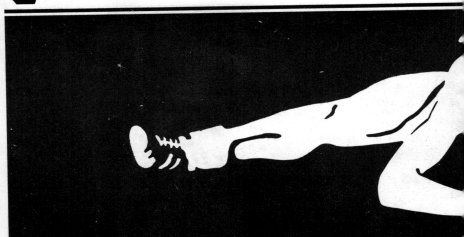

THERE IS ANOTHER WAY

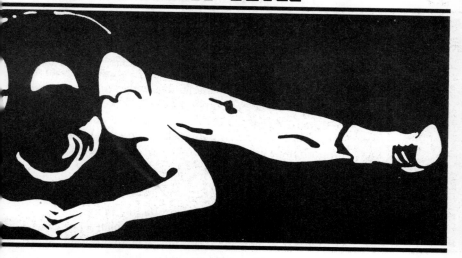

D EVELOPING FULL POTENTIAL

High-level fitness not only includes physiological components but those that relate to sociological and psychological growth and development as well. Since the human being is a complex organism living in a sophisticated environment it is essential that he develop within reason all of his potentialities. To do so, he should not rely on only one method for conditioning. Games, sports, hobbies, and other recreational activities should definitely become a part of everyone's life style.

Concomitant Learning. Participation in a variety of sports provides numerous opportunities for total fitness. It not only allows an opportunity for the development and maintenance of physical fitness, but at the same time provides a chance to increase mental and social skills. We need to be concerned with total development.

Wisdom versus Knowledge. Knowledge about the values derived from specific exercise should serve as a basic stimulus for increasing activity. But it is the assimilated wisdom flowing from its acquisition that tends to promote the greatest growth. Knowledge is the state of knowing, wisdom implies discerning behavior. The wise man will make use of the knowledge he possesses.

The Neutral Zone. Many of us are neither well nor sick; we are in the neutral zone. We fail to realize the unproductiveness of our existence. It is like being on a ship moving in many directions at the same time; it is like taking one step forward and sliding three feet backward. Not only is our physical development impeded, but so is our social, mental and spiritual growth. As we are assigned to a specific time slot in life, it behooves us to grow as much as possible in every conceivable way. Most of us fail to reach our potential. The quality of life is as important as its length. You do not have to be sick to get better.

QUALITY OF LIFE

This is a term used to describe the degree of competence, or grade of excellence, which a person is capable of achieving. Sports and activity programs afford many opportunities for qualitative living. The following examples are but a few of those available to the participant.

1. *Self-appraisal.* It doesn't take forever to appraise your ability in sports. You may evaluate yourself against others, or against established measurements and scores. In either instance, you have an opportunity to assess your strength and weakness. Furthermore, sports provide an easy opportunity to participate in enjoyable activities in which your measurements may be reviewed as you extend yourself. Eventually, a man should be able to accept himself for what he really is. A true assessment

makes known his actual status. Now we have an option: we can learn to live with it, or do something about it; the choice is ours.

2. *Taking the initiative.* If we are displeased with our status we can make an effort for change. Only we can control our own betterment; no one else can do it for us. It requires commitment and effort to improve physical, mental and social skills. Once this has been done, effective progress may be measured in numerous categories.

3. *Enthusiasm.* Interest, excitement, or eagerness about what we do tends to promote a greater effort; for some reason or other it seems to make our endeavors more worthwhile. Furthermore, enthusiasm is said to be contagious. Once it becomes a part of your own life style, the easier it will be for you to influence others. Try it out on someone—see if it doesn't work! Be responsible for stimulating others to be more active.

4. *Personality improvement.* Personality is defined as the pattern of collective character, behavior, temperament, emotional and mental traits of an individual. In essence, it portrays how we impress others and in return how they impress us.

   An individual's personality is enhanced by his health, enthusiasm, efforts, sportsmanship, and energy. These can be improved while participating in a worthwhile activity program. It behooves us to make the most favorable impression possible—it is another way of forging ahead in life.

5. *Understanding others.* It is a difficult task to understand others. Countless personal traits are revealed when we play. If concerned about the commitment, enthusiasm, honesty, and physical development of another, observe how he plays. Keep in mind that others can assess you in the same way.

6. *Friendly universe.* Life is too short to assume that the world is against us. Games, sports and play should be on a friendly basis. Never develop the attitude that you must win at all cost. This unhealthy

idea could permeate your entire life style. Remember the advice on the old locker-room poster—"It matters not who wins the game, but how the game was played." Rules are made so that the participants may have a safe, enjoyable, equal opportunity. Praise your opponent and he in return will have something nice to say about you.

7. *Be Optimistic.* The first step toward defeat is lack of confidence in your own ability. The old saying "Those that won't be beat, can't be beat" is often true in sports. Think you can make the shot, know you can execute the play—it's magic. The song, "Accentuate the Positive, Eliminate the Negative" represents an excellent attitude to develop about your performance. Keeping those thoughts in mind will help you win games you might otherwise have lost. Even if you do lose, there is always another time; prepare yourself for the coming contest.

8. *Be agreeable and friendly.* Few enjoy playing with a poor loser. Neither a whining, defensive cry-baby nor a grouchy, ill-humored participant makes many friends. "Smile and the world will smile with you; cry, and you cry alone." Don't get in the habit of fussing over other people's mistakes—they did not try to miss the putt!

9. *Elevate your goals.* Continuous improvement should be the goal. Never settle for your present physical, social, or mental status in life. Few people come close to their potential—we can improve tremendously in every respect. All that is necessary is to elevate our goals, and try harder to succeed. Never settle for second if first is possible.

10. *There is no defeat.* You may fail to get the highest score—but remember that the score is the smallest reason for participating in recreation and sports. The real purpose is to get exercise, develop endurance, strength, flexibility, and take advantage of the other benefits described in this book. If you are disturbed because you were outscored, you probably have a poor attitude. Remember, the score is of minimal importance in relation to all the values derived from being a participant.

ANOTHER WAY

Yes, there is another way to spend your leisure time besides doing nothing. Analyze your needs, then select a course of action through which these needs can be met. After selecting some activities to enhance your life style, establish a scheduled routine and follow it faithfully. You will improve your physical, social, mental and spiritual life. Our status in life depends to a significant degree upon the energy we are willing to expend; the dividends from living an active life are unequaled in any other life style.

LIFETIME SPORTS

There are many lifetime sports that may be used in the development and maintenance of total fitness. Not only do they contribute to physical conditioning, but to social and emotional well-being too. These sports provide an opportunity for the release of pent-up emotions, and at the same time enable you to build lifelong friendships with people with interests similar to yours.

When you choose the activities you wish to incorporate into your life style, keep in mind that certain activities may contribute more than others. Therefore, based on other conditions such as your work, size, weight and health, select those activities that would be most beneficial for you.

Activities that contribute to cardiorespiratory fitness are:

Badminton	Racquetball
Basketball	Skating (speed)
Bicycling	Skiing
(speed or hill)	(cross country)
Canoeing	Squash
Dancing (fast)	Surfing
Fencing	Swimming
Handball	Tennis
Jogging	Volleyball

Activities suitable for the development and maintenance of strength, endurance and flexibility are:

Calisthenics	Skating
Canoeing	(ice or roller)
Dancing	Skiing
Golf (carry your own clubs)	Skin Diving

Handball
Hiking (4-5 miles)
Jogging or running
Squash

Surfing
Swimming
Weight lifting

There are countless chores and amusements that may be included in your life style and which will contribute to total fitness. Some examples are:

Building an addition to your house
Camping (wilderness)
Chopping or sawing wood
Club activities
Entertaining friends
Gardening
Helping a neighbor with a work project
Hunting or fishing
Mowing and edging the lawn
Painting your house
Polishing the car
Scrubbing the floor
Walking to the market
Working on car or boat
Whistling, singing, playing a harmonica

Pleasant, money-saving, energy-consuming activities can really make life more enjoyable; if they are not now a part of your life, build them in. Above all, don't let your future be clouded by awareness of a gap between your fitness level and the level you wished to reach—start to close that gap now—and have fun!

SUGGESTED READINGS

Allen, T. Earl; Byrd, Ronald J.; and Smith, Douglas P. "Hemodynamic Consequences of Circuit Weight Training." *Research Quarterly:* October, 1976.

Allsen, Philip E.; Harrison, Joyce M.; and Vance, Barbara. *Fitness for Life.* Dubuque, Iowa: Wm. C. Brown Company Publishers. 1976.

Anderson, James L. and Cohen, Martin. *The Westpoint Fitness and Diet Book.* New York: Rawson Associates Publishers, Inc., 1977.

Clarke, David H. *Exercise Physiology.* Englewood Cliffs, New Jersey: Prentice-Hall, Inc., 1975.

SUGGESTED READINGS *(Con't.)*

Cooper, Kenneth H., et al. "An Aerobics Conditioning Program for the Fort Worth, Texas School District." *Research Quarterly:* October, 1975.

Crouch, James E. *Functional Human Anatomy.* Philadelphia: Lea and Febiger, 1967.

Cureton, Kirk J.; Boileau, Richard A.; and Lohman, Timothy A. "Relationship Between Body Composition Measures and AAHPER Test Performances in Young Boys." *Research Quarterly:* May, 1975.

Davis, Elwood Craig, et al. *Quality of Living.* Dubuque, Iowa: Wm. C. Brown Company Publishers, 1967.

Dawson, Helen L. *Basic Human Anatomy.* New York: Appleton-Century-Crofts, 1966.

Edington, D.W. and Cunningham, Lee. *Biological Awareness.* Englewood Cliffs, New Jersey: Prentice-Hall, Inc., 1975.

Falls, H.B.; Wallis, E.L.; and Logan, G.A. *Foundations of Conditioning.* New York: Academic Press, 1970.

Fixx, James F. *The Complete Book of Running.* New York: Random House, 1977.

Getchell, Bud. *Physical Fitness: A Way of Life.* New York: John Wiley and Sons, Inc., 1976.

Guild, Warren R. *How to Keep Fit and Enjoy It.* New York: Harper and Brothers, Publishers, 1962.

Hall, J. Tillman, et al. *Fundamentals of Physical Education.* Pacific Palisades, California: Goodyear Publishing Company, Inc., 1969.

Hall, J. Tillman; Sweeny, Nancy; and Esser, Jody. *Until the Whistle Blows.* Santa Monica, California: Goodyear Publishing Company, 1977.

Healy, Colin. *Methods of Fitness.* London: Kaye and Ward, 1973.

Hockey, Robert V. *Physical Fitness.* Saint Louis: The C.V. Mosby Company, 1977.

Holland, George J. and Davis, Elwood Craig. *Values of Physical Activity.* Dubuque, Iowa: Wm. C. Brown Company Publishers, 1975.

Hutton, Robert S., ed. *Exercise and Sport Sciences Reviews,* Vol. 5 Santa Barbara, California: Journal Publishing Affiliates, 1977.

Johnson, Warren, ed. *Science and Medicine of Exercise and Sport.* New York: Harper and Brothers Publishers, 1960.

Karpovich, Peter V. and Sinning, Wayne. *Physiology of Muscular Activity.* Philadelphia: W.B. Saunders Company, 1971.

Lawther, John D. *The Learning of Physical Skills.* Englewood Cliffs, New Jersey: Prentice-Hall, Inc., 1968.

SUGGESTED READINGS *(Con't.)*

Lindsey, Ruth; Jones, Billie J.; and Whitley, Ada Van.
Body Mechanics.
Dubuque, Iowa: Wm. C. Brown Company Publishers, 1979.

Logan, Gene A. and Dunkelberg, James G. *Adaptations of Muscular Activity.*
Belmont, California: Wadsworth Publishing Company, 1965.

Mathews, Donald K. *Measurement in Physical Education*
Philadelphia: W.B. Saunders Company, 1978.

Mathews, Donald K. and Fox, Edward L. *The Physiological Basis of Physical Education and Athletics.*
Philadelphia: W.B. Saunders Company, 1971.

Miller, Doris I. and Nelson, Richard. *Biomechanics of Sport.*
Philadelphia: Lea and Febiger, 1973.

Mott, Jane A. *Conditioning and Basic Movement Concepts.*
Dubuque, Iowa: Wm. C. Brown Company Publishers, 1977.

Nourse, Alan E. and the Editors of Life. *The Body.*
New York: Time Incorporated, 1964.

Pollock, Michael L.; Wilmore, Jack H.; and Fox III, Samuel M.
Health and Fitness Through Physical Activity.
New York: John Wiley and Sons, 1978.

President's Council on Physical Fitness. *Adult Physical Fitness.*
Washington, D.C.: U.S. Government Printing Office, 1978.

Rasch, Philip J. *Weight Training.*
Dubuque, Iowa: Wm. C. Brown Company, Publishers, 1979.

Ricci, Benjamin. *Physiological Basis of Human Performance.*
Philadelphia: Lea and Febiger, 1967.

Robb, Margaret D. *The Dynamics of Motor-Skill Acquisition.*
Englewood Cliffs, New Jersey: Prentice-Hall, Inc., 1972.

Selye, Hans. *The Stress of Life.*
New York: McGraw-Hill Book Company, Inc., 1956.

Sorani, Robert P. *Circuit Training.*
Dubuque, Iowa: Wm. C. Brown Company Publishers, 1966.

Stallings, Loretta M. *Motor Skills.*
Dubuque, Iowa: Wm. C. Brown Company Publishers, 1973.

Sweigard, Lulu E. *Human Movement Potential.*
New York: Dodd Mead and Company, 1974.

Van Huss, Wayne D., et al. *Physical Activity in Modern Living.*
Englewood Cliffs, New Jersey: Prentice-Hall, Inc., 1969.

Vitale, Frank. *Individualized Fitness Programs.*
Englewood Cliffs, New Jersey: Prentice-Hall, Inc., 1973.

Wilmore, Jack H. *Athletic Training and Physical Fitness.*
Boston: Allyn and Bacon, Inc., 1976.

Wilmore, Jack H., ed. *Exercise and Sport Sciences Reviews.*
Vol. 1.
New York: Academic Press, 1973.

Wilmore, Jack H., ed. *Exercise and Sport Sciences Reviews.*
Vol. 2.
New York: Academic Press, 1974.

PERIODICALS

Aronchick, Joel and Burke, Edmund. "Psycho-Physical Effects of Varied Rest Intervals Following Warm-Up."
Research Quarterly: May, 1977.

Astrand, Per-Olaf. *Health and Fitness.*
New York: Barron's-Woodbury, 1977.

Barrow, Harold M. *Man and Movement: Principles of Physical Education.*
Philadelphia: Lea and Febiger, 1977.

Baumgartner, Ted A. and Zuidema, Marvin A. "Factor Analysis of Physical Fitness Tests."
Research Quarterly: December, 1972.

Boileau, Richard A.; Massey, Benjamin H.; and Misner, James E. "Body Composition Changes in Adult Men During Selected Weight Training and Jogging Programs."
Research Quarterly: May, 1973.

Bonner, Hugh W. "Preliminary Exercise: A Two Factor Theory."
Research Quarterly: May, 1974.

Burke, Edmund J. "Validity of Selected Laboratory and Field Tests of Physical Working Capacity."
Research Quarterly: March, 1976.

Foster, Carl. "Physiological Requirements of Aerobic Dancing."
Research Quarterly: March, 1975.

Hinson, Marilyn and Rosentswieg, Joel. "Comparative Electromyographic Values of Isometric, Isotonic, and Isokinetic Contraction."
Research Quarterly: December, 1972.

Katch, Victor; Weltman, Arthur; and Traeger, Laurel. "All-Out Versus a Steady-Paced Cycling Strategy for Maximal Work Output of Short Duration."
Research Quarterly: May, 1976.

Katch, Victor L. and Katch, Frank I. "Reliability, Individual Differences and Intravariation of Endurance Performance on the Bicycle Ergometer."
Research Quarterly: March, 1972.

Laurie, David R. Jr. "Live Lecture Versus Slide-Tape Method of Instruction for a Health Unit of Physical Fitness."
Research Quarterly: December, 1976.

Lloyd, Andrew J. "Auditory EMG Feedback During a Sustained Submaximum Isometric Contraction."
Research Quarterly: March, 1972.

Marley, William P. and Tennerud, Ardell C. "A Three-Year Study of the Astrand-Rhyming Step Test."
Research Quarterly: May, 1976.

McCafferty, William B. and Horvath, Steven M. "Specificity of Exercise and Specificity of Training: A Subcellular Review."
Research Quarterly: May, 1977.

McKinney, Donald, et al. "Investigation of a Training Shoe as a Supplemental Conditioning Device."

PERIODICALS *(Con't.)*

Research Quarterly: May 1975.

Moffatt, Robert J.; Stamford, Bryant A.; and Neill, Robert D. "Placement of Tri-Weekly Training Sessions: Importance Regarding Enhancement of Aerobic Capacity." *Research Quarterly:* October, 1977.

Montoye, Henry J., et al. "Fitness, Fatness and Serum Cholesterol: An Epidermiological Study of an Entire Community." *Research Quarterly:* October, 1976.

Morris, Alfred F. "Effects of Fatiguing Isometric and Isotonic Exercise on Fractionated Patellar Tendon Reflex Components." *Research Quarterly:* March, 1977.

Noble, Larry and McCraw, Lynn W. "Comparative Effects of Isometric and Isotonic Training Programs on Relative Endurance and Work Capacity." *Research Quarterly:* December, 1972.

Pollock, Michael L.; Broida, Jeffrey; and Kendrick, Zebulon. "Validity of the Palpation Technique of Heart Rate Determination and its Estimation of Training Heart Rate." *Research Quarterly:* March, 1972.

Shaver, Larry G. "Relation of Maximum Isometric Strength and Relative Isotonic Endurance of the Elbow Flexors of Athletes." *Research Quarterly:* March, 1972.

Sparling, Phillip B. "Exercise Stress Testing Programs in the United States: A 1975 Status Study." *Research Quarterly:* December, 1977.

Vodack, Paul A. and Wilmore, Jack H. "Validity of the 6-Minute Jog-Walk and the 600 Yard Run-Walk in Estimating Endurance Capacity in Boys 9-12 Years." *Research Quarterly:* May, 1975.

Wiley, Jack F. and Shaver, Larry G. "Prediction of Maximum Oxygen Intake from Running Performances of Untrained Young Men." *Research Quarterly:* March, 1972.

Young, R. John and Ismail, A. H. "Comparison of Selected Physiological and Personality Variables in Regular and Non-Regular Adult Male Exercisers." *Research Quarterly:* October, 1977.

Young, R. John and Ismail, A. H. "Personality Differences of Adult Men Before and After a Physical Fitness Program." *Research Quarterly:* October, 1976.

Zingale, Donald P. " 'Ike' Revisited on Sport and National Fitness." *Research Quarterly:* March, 1977.

Zuidma, Marvin A. and Baumgartner, Ted A. "Second Factor Analysis Study of Physical Fitness Tests." *Research Quarterly:* October, 1974.

PHYSICAL FITNESS PROFILE

(Self testing—Easy to do—See how you change)

Date									
Height									
Weight									
ENDURANCE: Step Test Score									
Rope Skipping									
Two Mile Run									
STRENGTH: Number Chin-ups									
Number Push-ups									
Number Sit-ups									
FLEXIBILITY: Bend and Reach									
Sit and Reach									
HOURS YOU EXERCISE PER WEEK									

FLEXIBILITY INDICATOR

Date _____ Height _____ Weight _____

	Time spent on exercise	Number of repititions
Bend and Stretch		
Wing Stretch		
Body Bender		
Ankle Stretch		
Sitting Stretch		
Toe Touch		
Knee-to-Head Stretch		
Achilles Stretch		
Leg Over		
Bench Stretch		
Sitting Curl		
Monkey Roll		
Back Rocker		
Side Stretcher		
Chair Stretcher		
Elevated Curl-Ups		
Pull Stretcher		
Bend and Reach		
Sit and Reach		
Trunk Extension		

PHYSICAL FITNESS PROFILE

(Self testing—Easy to do—See how you change)

Date										
Height										
Weight										
ENDURANCE: Step Test Score										
Rope Skipping										
Two Mile Run										
STRENGTH: Number Chin-ups										
Number Push-ups										
Number Sit-ups										
FLEXIBILITY: Bend and Reach										
Sit and Reach										
HOURS YOU EXERCISE PER WEEK										

PHYSICAL FITNESS PROFILE

(Self testing—Easy to do—See how you change)

Date											
Height											
Weight											
ENDURANCE: Step Test Score											
Rope Skipping											
Two Mile Run											
STRENGTH: Number Chin-ups											
Number Push-ups											
Number Sit-ups											
FLEXIBILITY: Bend and Reach											
Sit and Reach											
HOURS YOU EXERCISE PER WEEK											

PHYSICAL FITNESS PROFILE

(Self testing—Easy to do—See how you change)

Date										
Height										
Weight										
ENDURANCE: Step Test Score										
Rope Skipping										
Two Mile Run										
STRENGTH: Number Chin-ups										
Number Push-ups										
Number Sit-ups										
FLEXIBILITY: Bend and Reach										
Sit and Reach										
HOURS YOU EXERCISE PER WEEK										

FLEXIBILITY INDICATOR

Date _____ Height _____ Weight _____

	Time spent on exercise	Number of repititions
Bend and Stretch		
Wing Stretch		
Body Bender		
Ankle Stretch		
Sitting Stretch		
Toe Touch		
Knee-to-Head Stretch		
Achilles Stretch		
Leg Over		
Bench Stretch		
Sitting Curl		
Monkey Roll		
Back Rocker		
Side Stretcher		
Chair Stretcher		
Elevated Curl-Ups		
Pull Stretcher		
Bend and Reach		
Sit and Reach		
Trunk Extension		

FLEXIBILITY INDICATOR

Date _____ Height _____ Weight _____

	Time spent on exercise	Number of repititions
Bend and Stretch		
Wing Stretch		
Body Bender		
Ankle Stretch		
Sitting Stretch		
Toe Touch		
Knee-to-Head Stretch		
Achilles Stretch		
Leg Over		
Bench Stretch		
Sitting Curl		
Monkey Roll		
Back Rocker		
Side Stretcher		
Chair Stretcher		
Elevated Curl-Ups		
Pull Stretcher		
Bend and Reach		
Sit and Reach		
Trunk Extension		

FLEXIBILITY INDICATOR

Date _____ Height _____ Weight _____

	Time spent on exercise	Number of repititions
Bend and Stretch		
Wing Stretch		
Body Bender		
Ankle Stretch		
Sitting Stretch		
Toe Touch		
Knee-to-Head Stretch		
Achilles Stretch		
Leg Over		
Bench Stretch		
Sitting Curl		
Monkey Roll		
Back Rocker		
Side Stretcher		
Chair Stretcher		
Elevated Curl-Ups		
Pull Stretcher		
Bend and Reach		
Sit and Reach		
Trunk Extension		